MW00463356

ENERGY HEALING

for

Relationships

About the Authors

Sabine and Keith have more than thirty years of experience working with individuals and families in North America, Europe, and Africa. In addition to the techniques they personally developed, they've drawn inspiration and technical knowledge from ancient Yoga, Tantra, Taoism, and Chinese Medicine, as well as modern scientific research into nutrition, family constellations, and parenting.

Keith Sherwood is a master of the four classical Yogas. He is the author of nine books on energy work, healing, and transcendent relationship. The exercises, mudras, and meditations that he has developed are used throughout Europe and North America by healers and energy practitioners to heal physical disease, deep traumas, karmic wounds, and energetic blockages. His ability to see and analyze subtle fields of energy and consciousness has been instrumental in helping people achieve their spiritual goals.

Sabine Wittmann was born in Salzburg, Austria, and graduated from Heilpraktiker (Natural Healer) School in Munich, Germany. In 1997, she opened a private practice for energy healing in Berlin. She has been giving lectures and seminars, as well as writing articles, in Germany, Austria, and Turkey for more than ten years. In 2014, she co-authored *Energy Healing for Women*, which was published by Llewellyn Worldwide.

Sabine currently specializes in women's issues, focusing particularly on the psychological and energetic issues surrounding fertility. As a practitioner of energy work, homeopathy, and several whole-body therapies, she has seen firsthand how conditioning and subtle cultural prejudices still adversely affect the energetic and physical health of women. Her goal is to help modern women become more creative, radiant, joyful, and free.

Together, Keith and Sabine have created a holistic system that can enhance compatibility and demonstrate that family members have the innate power to overcome even the most divisive relationship patterns.

Through their timely intervention and ability to release distorted fields of energy and consciousness, Keith and Sabine have empowered parents and children who have struggled to nurture one another and achieve lasting intimate relationships. They've helped relationship partners overcome sexual patterns that have driven them apart. They've taught couples how to make decisions that were life-affirming and that enhanced family relationships.

And they've helped family members overcome trauma scars in their subtle field and energetic poisons that they inherited from their birth families and which, in this incarnation, have created self-limiting patterns that disrupt family relationships.

By using the information and techniques they've developed, you will be able to achieve deeper levels of communication, trust, and intimacy that you and your family members have wanted to experience but never thought were possible.

ENERGY
HEALING

for Relationships

·····················
Meditations, Mudras,
and Chakra Practices *for* Partners,
Families, and Friends
·············

Keith Sherwood
AND Sabine Wittmann

Llewellyn Publications
Woodbury, Minnesota

FIRST EDITION
First Printing, 2019

Cover design by Shira Atakpu
Editing by Holly Vanderhaar
Interior illustrations by Mary Ann Zapalac
Interior Mudra photos by Keith Sherwood

Llewellyn Publications is a registered trademark of Llewellyn Worldwide Ltd.

Library of Congress Cataloging-in-Publication Data (Pending)
ISBN: 978-0-7387-5206-8

Llewellyn Worldwide Ltd. does not participate in, endorse, or have any authority or responsibility concerning private business transactions between our authors and the public.
   All mail addressed to the author is forwarded but the publisher cannot, unless specifically instructed by the author, give out an address or phone number.
   Any internet references contained in this work are current at publication time, but the publisher cannot guarantee that a specific location will continue to be maintained. Please refer to the publisher's website for links to authors' websites and other sources.

Llewellyn Publications
A Division of Llewellyn Worldwide Ltd.
2143 Wooddale Drive
Woodbury, MN 55125-2989
www.llewellyn.com

Printed in the United States of America

Contents

Exercises

Chapter 14: Strengthening the Family Field

Chapter 15: Overcoming Parental Challenges

Chapter 16: Overcoming Internal Threats to the Family

Chapter 17: Overcoming External Threats to the Family

Chapter 18: Empty-Nesters

Illustrations

Introduction

Andrew and his first wife were divorced in 2002. Shortly after their divorce, Andrew's son and daughter refused to have any further contact with him. He was heartbroken, but eventually accepted their decision. Several years later, he remarried and to his dismay the pattern repeated itself with his two adult step-children. Although none of the children involved would have contact with him, they ultimately disclosed how they felt to their respective mothers, who shared what they'd heard with Andrew during the process of deep family healing.

According to both women, the crux of the problem was a huge blind spot that blocked Andrew's empathy and prevented him from caring for anyone but himself. To compound the problem, Andrew was unable to express any emotion except anger. To heal the family dynamic, we asked Andrew to reflect on what he'd heard—and to find out everything he could about the pattern, including how it developed and how it had influenced his family relationships. Andrew found this difficult to do because he had no experience reflecting on himself.

In an effort to help him, we taught him to create his own healing space and to center his awareness inside his body, soul, and spirit. From experience, we knew that this exercise could help him get in touch with his emotions. It would also make it easier for him to reflect on who he was and what motivated him to act the way he did. It was gratifying for us to see Andrew's progress and the changes he experienced once he began to perform the exercise.

In the next few chapters, you will learn how Andrew's family, and families like your own, healed their relationships and reconciled themselves with their family members. And you will learn how you can use the same techniques they did to overcome self-limiting patterns and enhance the joy and satisfaction you and your loved ones get from your family relationships.

Deep Family Healing is for Everyone

Deep family healing is for everyone. It doesn't matter who you are or what type of family you're in. If you want more from your family relationships, this is the right book for you. Even if there are cultural differences, religious differences—or you and your family members are separated by time and space—you can use this book to get more nourishment, strength, and satisfaction from your family relationships. In fact, from the information, tips, and exercises you will learn to perform in *Energy Healing for Relationships*, you will be able to transform your relationships by healing the wounds, blockages, and attachments that drive family members apart at their root, in your subtle field of energy and consciousness.

In *Energy Healing for Relationships*, we will share our experiences and the experiences of the people we've worked with, who—like yourselves—have striven to create more joyful and enduring family relationships. This book is dedicated to enhancing the well-being of all family members and to ensuring that children are empowered and grow up with all the love and self-confidence they need to succeed in their adult life. For us, the well-being of children has always come first.

Challenging Times

It doesn't take a sage to know that in the modern world, families of all types face many challenges—some old, some new. Family relationships can be disrupted, and family members can be pulled apart.

There are many ways that these things can happen. Relatives and friends can interfere with family relationships. Social media can interfere with a parent's natural authority or the natural development of a child's character. Some parents can use their children to compensate for their limitations—and partners can become so overwhelmed by the needs of their children that they end up with no space within themselves to enjoy their life or family relationships.

Our book addresses these challenges and more. In *Energy Healing for Relationships* we've provided readers with an easy-to-implement system of deep healing that is accessible to all family members. Our system works because it focuses on the real issues families face and it heals family relationships—not just individuals—on the deepest levels of energy and consciousness.

In *Energy Healing for Relationships*, readers will learn to recognize and release attachments that can interfere with communication, understanding, and the harmony of family members. The attachments we're referring to are not limited by time-space. They are actual structures that, in the form of non-physical fields and blockages, can keep people connected to one another from one lifetime to another.

Our system of deep healing has been thirty years in the making. In that time, we've learned that it's essential for family members to take control of their healing and spiritual development. Fortunately, the people we've worked with, who accepted that responsibility, quickly recognized that their family members served as mirrors that reflected their personal issues back to them. They also recognized that there was nothing fundamentally wrong with them. All they needed was a system of deep family healing that could make the aspirations they had for themselves and their family a reality.

Even if you or one of your family members are skeptical—or if you think you can never forgive yourself or a family member for an injury that took place on the physical and/or subtle levels—you can use what you learn in this book to heal the wounds that have interfered with the love and intimacy that are the basis of family relationships. If you're ready, you can begin the process of deep family healing, like Andrew, by creating your own personal healing space.

EXERCISE: Personal Healing Space

Your personal healing space is a place without limitations where you can tap into your discernment and dormant healing power. It's a place where communication and understanding supplant self-limiting beliefs and patterns. Once you've created your personal healing space, you can use it along with the other exercises you will learn to perform in this book to heal yourself and your relationships on the levels of body, soul, and spirit.

When you're ready to begin, sit in a quiet place where you won't be disturbed by other people or digital devices. Bring your awareness to your physical-material body. Enjoy its sensations for two to three minutes. Then bring your awareness to your soul. Your soul contains your authentic feelings, emotions, and your authentic mind. Like your physical-material body, it will emerge as a field which adds to your complete experience of the world inside and outside you.

Take two to three minutes to enjoy your soul. Then bring your awareness to your spirit. Since your spirit transcends feelings and emotions, you won't feel your spirit. But you can experience it through your awareness, empathy, and unconditional love. Take two to three minutes to experience your spirit. Then take ten more minutes to enjoy the effects the process has had on your subtle field and physical-material body.

By performing this exercise regularly, you will quickly recognize that you have unlimited resources of power, joy, and love that you can use to heal family dynamics.

Energy Healing for Relationships has been divided into six parts. In each part, we have focused on family dynamics and the issues that bear directly on the health and well-being of long-term, intimate relationships and parenting. Since you can't separate personal well-being from healthy family relationships, we've included accounts of families that will illustrate how deep family healing can enhance the joy and satisfaction that family members experience with one another.

In part 1, you will learn how your non-physical field of energy and consciousness interacts with the physical and non-physical world and how subtle forces can drive family members apart. We will look at several families and how they healed their family relationships. Like them, you will learn to enhance your level of energy and consciousness. We've provided you with exercises that will center your awareness in your non-physical field—and enhance your empathy for yourself and your family.

In part 2, we will explain how your soul vibration, core values, and the balance of elements in your subtle field and physical-material body influence your choice of a life partner—and the health of your relationships.

Choosing an appropriate life partner is one of the most important decisions you will make. In part 2, you will learn to enhance your inner wisdom and use muscle testing to choose a partner who is the right fit for you and your lifestyle. If you're already in a long-term, intimate relationship, you can use the exercises we've provided to harmonize your soul vibration, core values, and dominant element with those of your partner so that you experience more joy in your relationship.

In part 3, you will learn to make a seamless transition from single life to family life. And you will learn to create the Mutual Field of Prana—so that you can share life-affirming energy effortlessly with your partner. We've identified a number of disruptive life-patterns in part 3 that can interfere with even the most loving family relationships. We will explain how these patterns develop, how partners can avoid them and, when necessary, how partners can heal them.

The five elements—earth, wood, metal, water, and fire—provide structure and stability to your life and relationships. In part 3, we will provide you with exercises designed to strengthen weak elements. By strengthening them you will empower yourself and make your relationships more stable.

In part 4, you will learn how you and your partner can prepare yourselves for the arrival of children. We've provided you with exercises to increase the amount of space you have within your subtle field of energy and consciousness. By creating more space, you will be able to share your feelings and emotions effortlessly with your partner and children. Expectant mothers will learn to enhance the health of their non-physical field as well as the energetic condition of their pre-born. We've included exercises to enlarge the mutual field of prana to include children and to heal birth traumas and common childhood ailments that have their foundation in your newborn's subtle field.

In part 5, we've provided you with tips and techniques designed to help your child flourish both at home and in school. You will learn to fill your pre-schooler's subtle field with chi (prana) and to strengthen your children's wood element, which is the dominant element for all preschool children. We have also provided you with energetic solutions for some of the most common problems faced by preschoolers, including bedwetting, thumb-sucking, sleep problems, etc.

In part 5, special attention has been given to specific challenges you and your loved ones may face in the modern world, including gender and sexual development, depression, body image problems, violence, and character development. Since ancestral poisons and karmic baggage can inhibit a child's development and a parent's well-being, we've provided you with simple techniques to release the blockages they've created.

In part 5, you will also learn how to let your grown children go, at the appropriate time, by creating the Mutual Field of Empathy and by performing the Radiant Tao Meditation. These exercises are designed to release unhealthy attachments so that even after your grown children have left the nest, all of you will remain close to one another and continue to share love effortlessly.

Empty-nesters face their own challenges. With that in mind, we've provided them with exercises to help them to grow old joyfully, and to overcome resentment and regret.

PART 1
You're an Inter-Dimensional Being

In part 1, you will be introduced to your non-physical field of energy and consciousness. You will learn simple exercises designed to liberate the immense amount of energy and consciousness you have available to heal yourself and your family relationships. Those of you familiar with our work will recognize some of these exercises. In *Energy Healing for Relationships*, they serve as the foundation of more advanced techniques designed specifically to overcome patterns and blockages that interfere with compatibility, family relationships, and early childhood development.

— ONE —
The Subtle Field of Energy and Consciousness

For those of you ready to transform your family relationships, it's important to recognize that family life can be a source of strength, joy, and fulfillment for all family members. Not only does family life elicit deep feelings of love and empathy, but also the demands of family life require that parents transcend their limits by enhancing their self-knowledge, self-control, empathy, honesty, selflessness, and respect for the feelings and needs of others, particularly their children.

For a growing child, family is where the soul begins its journey on earth. A healthy family life is the foundation on which character, self-esteem, health, happiness, and success are built and find support. The family and its relationships are the model for all the child's subsequent relationships, including their relationships to themselves, to other people, to work, leisure, and parenting. Therefore, it's important to recognize that family members interact in both a physical-material and subtle world of energy and consciousness; and that interactions on the subtle levels have as much or more influence on family dynamics and the quality of family relationships as interactions on the physical-material plane. It's also important to recognize that every human being is an inter-dimensional being who has a physical-material body and a subtle field of energy and consciousness that interpenetrates it.

Like an electrical grid that provides energy to homes and businesses, your subtle (non-physical) field provides you with all the energy and consciousness you need to function healthfully, to participate in intimate family relationships, and to perform deep healing.

The ancient adepts of both Yoga and Taoism taught that your non-physical field manifests as both a field of pure, life-affirming consciousness and a field of energy with universal qualities.

In Yoga, pure consciousness is called *prajnana* or *vijnana*, and non-physical energy is called *prana*. In Taoism, consciousness is known as the *Dao*, which manifests as awareness, perception, and bliss. Life-affirming energy is divided into three related forms. *Chi* (prana) represents the essential energy or life force, while *jing* represents its essence—how it is manifest in your life. The third essential element is the spirit or original form of the energy. In this book, you will learn to use both consciousness in its purest form and non-physical energy along with its essence to heal yourself and your family relationships.

In addition to consciousness and energy, you have vehicles and organs of consciousness and energy in your subtle field. They go by various names including chakras, auras, dantians, etc. The purpose of these vehicles and organs is to process all the consciousness and energy in your subtle field—so that you can form a life-affirming identity and share your ideas, emotions, and feelings joyfully with the people you love.

Unfortunately, both consciousness and energy with universal qualities can be blocked. And it's blockages—and the restrictive patterns they create—that explain why, even with all the consciousness and energy people have available, many of them still have difficulty reaching their potential and creating the joyful family relationships they desire. In spite of all this, we are convinced that, by using the information and practicing the exercises in this book, you can release blockages in your subtle field and create a new reality for yourself and your family.

To do this, you will utilize a kit of easy-to-use tools that will allow you to observe the condition of your subtle field and release distorted fields of energy and consciousness that have been interfering with your family relationships.

You already learned to use your awareness to create your personal healing space. In this chapter, you will be introduced to two additional tools which—

like awareness—will make healing your family relationships easier than you think. The tools we're referring to are your intent and mental attention.

It's the simplicity of our system and its toolkit which has inspired so many people, even those who were skeptical at first, to commit themselves to healing their family relationships. By using your intent and mental attention along with your personal healing space in a systematic way, in a short time you will be able to overcome self-limiting patterns and heal the relationships that are most dear to you.

How to Use the Intent

In deep family healing, your intent serves the same function as a computer software program. Just as a software program instructs a computer to perform a particular task, your intent will instruct your authentic mind, which is composed of your brain, central nervous system, and your non-physical field of energy and consciousness, to perform healing on both the physical and subtle levels of energy and consciousness. Your intent is one of your most useful functions of mind. And if you use your intent properly—without watching yourself, trying too hard, or mixing your intent with sentiment and self-doubt—it will become a valuable tool that you will use in virtually all the healing techniques contained within this book.[1]

How to Use the Mental Attention

Your mental attention is another function of mind that can have a profound effect on your personal well-being and the well-being of your family relationships. By using your mental attention skillfully, you can bring all of your innate powers to bear on any part of your subtle field and physical-material body. That's because your mental attention functions simultaneously in all worlds and dimensions in both the physical and non-physical universe. With the intent as a guide, your mental attention can be used to heal even the most divisive and resistant patterns that have pulled you and your family members apart.[2]

We recommend that you strengthen your intent and mental attention before you begin to use them to heal your family relationships. You can begin to strengthen your intent by using it to bring more joy into your life.

To do that, find a place where you won't be disturbed. Then sit down, close your eyes, and breathe deeply through your nose for two to three minutes. When you're relaxed, assert, *"It's my intent to feel more joyful."* Then wait. If you don't interfere with the process, you may be surprised at how quickly your soul and spirit respond to your instructions. Of course, the process won't work if you attempt to use your intent to make yourself taller or shorter—because that's not something either your soul or spirit can do. And it won't work if you watch yourself, try too hard, or mix your intent with self-doubt or desires that emerge from your ego. But it will work if you instruct your soul and spirit to do something they can realistically do. That means you can use your intent to become more patient, more disciplined, more understanding, and/or more intuitive. And of course, you can use your intent to heal yourself and your family relationships.

As your confidence in the process grows, you can begin to use your intent along with your mental attention to activate pleasure centers in your physical-material body and subtle field and center yourself in them. Two pleasure centers that can be easily activated by your intent and mental attention are your human heart and Atman, the thumb sized point on the right side of your chest, where bliss enters your conscious awareness (see figure 1: The Three Hearts, page 13).

Activating Your Human Heart

To use your intent and mental attention to activate your human heart, sit in a comfortable position with your eyes closed. Then breathe deeply through your nose for two to three minutes. When you're relaxed, bring your mental attention to your human heart. The energetic center of your human heart is two inches (six centimeters) left of the middle point of your breastbone. Once your mental attention is centered, assert, *"It's my intent to activate my human heart."* Don't do anything after that. Just enjoy the process for as long as you want—because you can't go wrong by activating your human heart.

Activating Atman

In this exercise, you will activate and center yourself in Atman. Activating and centering yourself in Atman will be just as simple as activating your human heart. But the experience may be more intense because it's not human love that emerges from Atman—it's universal love. Since universal love is a form of consciousness, not energy, you can't feel it. Instead, you will probably experience it—at least in the beginning—as a buzz that radiates through your body—often from one body part to another. Sometimes, a sense of inner peace will begin to radiate through your subtle field and physical-material body once you've activated Atman and centered yourself in it because universal love is the solution to most of life's most enduring problems.

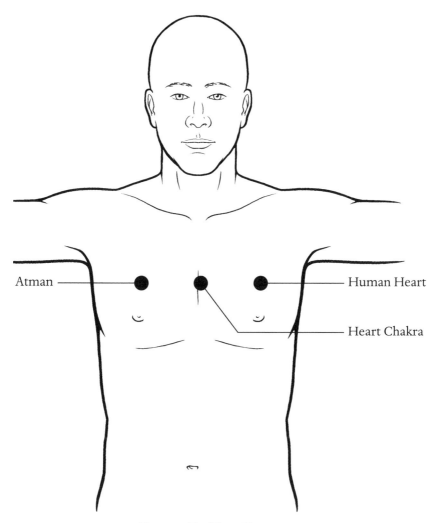

Figure 1: The Three Hearts

To activate and center yourself in Atman, sit in a comfortable position with your eyes closed. Then breathe deeply through your nose for two to three minutes. When you're relaxed, bring your mental attention to Atman; then assert, *"It's my intent to activate and center myself in Atman."* Don't do anything after that. Just enjoy the process for at least ten minutes or longer if you want— because you can't go wrong by activating and centering yourself in Atman.

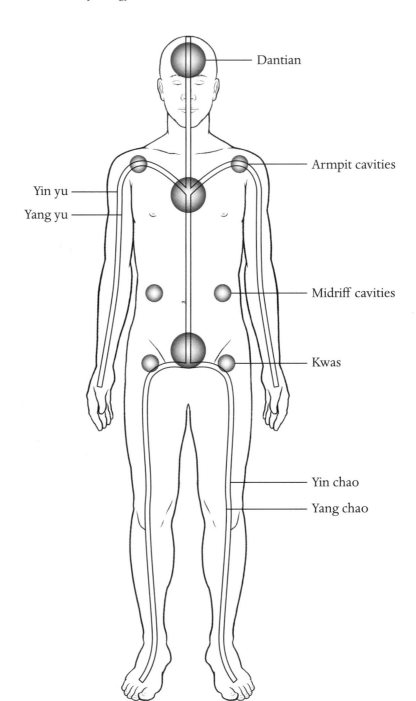

Figure 2: Taoist Subtle Anatomy

You can use these simple techniques to find inner peace whenever the stress of life interferes with your well-being.

Now that you are more familiar with your intent and mental attention, you can use them along with your personal healing space to supercharge your subtle field. You can do that by performing an exercise called the Golden Light Technique. It's based on the work of Taoist adepts, who were among the first people to address family issues on the subtle levels of energy and consciousness.

According to the Taoists, chi—a form of non-physical energy—was at the center of family life. Chi is identical to prana. When chi was able to flow freely, family members could share pleasure, love, intimacy, and joy with one another without restrictions. When it was blocked, relationships were disrupted because family members lost the capacity to empathize with one another and to express themselves freely.

The center of Taoist teaching was China. It was there in the sixth century BCE where the basic principles were laid out by Lao Tzu. Not much is known about his personal life—but we do know that, like his contemporaries in India, he taught that the physical-material world was the outer manifestation of a non-physical world of energy and consciousness that influenced all interactions that took place within it. According to Lao Tzu and the Taoist adepts that followed him, all this subtle energy and consciousness is processed by a human's subtle field, which consists of systems and organs designed specifically for that purpose. According to the Taoists, the subtle anatomy of a human being consists of energy centers (acupuncture points), channels of energy (meridians), and cavities that have various names and that serve as reservoirs of subtle energy and consciousness (see figure 2: Taoist Subtle Anatomy, page 14). Although we will delve more deeply into the anatomy of the subtle field later in this chapter, what is most important for us now are the three central reservoirs of energy described by Taoist adepts. From figure 2, you can see that the lowest reservoir is located in the center of the abdomen. It's called the lower dantian. Located above it, in the center of the chest, is the middle dantian, and located in the center of the head is the third reservoir, the upper dantian.

In the Golden Light Technique, you will increase the amount of chi you have available for all of your daily activities by enhancing the amount of chi you have stored in the three dantians. Having more chi available will do more than just energize you—it will enable you to express yourself more freely and share more activities with the people you love. It will enhance your motivation and fuel your creativity. And by performing the Golden Light Technique regularly, you will build up three reservoirs of energy with universal qualities that you can use to heal yourself and your loved ones.

EXERCISE: The Golden Light Technique

To perform the Golden Light Technique, find a comfortable position with your back straight. Then close your eyes and breathe deeply through your nose for two to three minutes. Deep nasal breathing will help you to relax. Once you're relaxed, assert in a normal voice, *"It's my intent to bring my mental attention to my lower dantian, in the center of my abdomen"* (see figure 2: Taoist Subtle Anatomy, page 14). Once your mental attention has been centered in your lower dantian for a few moments, bring your hands up to your chest and, with the palms facing each other, rub the tips of your corresponding fingers together until you feel a golden flame (chi) ignite in the center of your lower dantian. Experience the flame getting stronger until the lower dantian has been filled with its light. Take a few moments to enjoy the effects. Then remove your attention from your lower dantian and assert, *"It's my intent to bring my mental attention to my middle dantian, in the center of my chest."* Rub the tips of your corresponding fingers together again until you feel a golden flame ignite in the center of your middle dantian. Take a few moments to enjoy the effects— which should intensify as more chi becomes available. After you've removed your attention from your middle dantian, assert, *"It's my intent to bring my mental attention to my upper dantian, in the center of my head."* Rub the tips of your corresponding fingers together again until you feel a golden flame ignite in the center of your upper dantian. Take a few moments to enjoy the effects. Then complete the energetic circuit created by your subtle energy system by bringing the tip of your tongue to the back of your upper teeth and by putting the soles of your feet together. By completing the circuit, you will enhance the distribution of chi through the organs of your subtle field and physical-material body.

To continue, imagine that all the molecules of your body are being filled by this golden light—and that it expands until it surrounds you on all sides. Continue to float in this pool of chi for another ten minutes. Then return your tongue, feet, and hands to their normal position. After that, count from one to five. When you reach the number five, open your eyes and bring yourself out of the exercise.

We recommend that you practice the Golden Light Technique every other day, in the morning before you eat. By making it part of your regular regimen of deep healing and energy work, you will continue to increase the amount of energy that you can share with your loved ones.

The Visual Screen

Now that you've learned to use your intent and mental attention to perform the Golden Light Technique, you can use them along with your healing space to create a visual screen. A visual screen is a reliable tool that can be used to examine the condition of your subtle field or another person's subtle field—while you perform deep healing.

The visual screen you will create should be white and large enough to fit a life-sized image of a person. And it should be located eight feet (two and a half meters) in front of you and raised off the floor—so that you must look up at a thirty-degree angle to see the image on the screen clearly.

EXERCISE: The Visual Screen

To create a visual screen, find a comfortable position with your back straight. Close your eyes and breathe deeply through your nose for two to three minutes. Then count backward from five to one and from ten to one. Next, go to your personal healing space. Once you've brought your awareness to your body, soul, and spirit, assert, *"It's my intent to create a white screen eight feet (two and a half meters) in front of me."* Once the visual screen has materialized, assert, *"It's my intent to visualize an image of myself on the screen."* Immediately, you will see an image of yourself appear on the screen in a size to fit comfortably. Observe it for about five minutes. After five minutes, release the image of yourself and the visual screen. Then count from one to five. When you reach the number five, open your eyes and bring yourself out of the meditation.

We recommend that you practice this exercise every day until the screen appears immediately after you've programmed it to materialize—and you can see the image of yourself clearly.

Now that you've learned to enter your healing space and to use your intent and mental attention to create a visual screen, you're ready to use these three tools to take a journey through your subtle field.

Taking a journey through your subtle field will do two things. It will enhance your discernment, which is a form of intuition that healers use regularly to diagnose the condition of their client's subtle field. And it will give you valuable experience working on the non-physical levels of energy and consciousness.

We originally developed the journey for Petra, a thirty-one-year-old visual artist. She'd been practicing some of our techniques, but hadn't been able to heal a sleep issue that afflicted her three-year-old daughter Sarah. Whenever Petra tried to center herself and create a visual screen, her mind would wander and she would lose both her center and the screen before she could effectively perform the techniques of deep healing. In order to help her develop discernment and to stay centered, we developed the journey through the subtle field. We knew that this visually oriented journey would be effective for a visual artist—and within a short time, our intuition proved correct. Petra continued to make journeys through her subtle field until she perfected the technique. And within weeks of perfecting it, she was able to observe the organs of her subtle field and use the techniques of deep healing to heal her daughter.

Like Petra, in your journey through your subtle field, you will observe the dantians. It's interesting to note that Sarah's sleep problem was caused by a lack of chi in her lower dantian. In our work, we've learned that a lack of chi can lead to anxiety and excessive worry, both of which can make it difficult for a child to fall asleep and to sleep peacefully.

After you've observed the three dantians, you will proceed to examine six smaller reservoirs of chi located beside them. The lower two reservoirs are located on each side of the lower dantian and are connection to them. They are called the right and left kwas. Above them, located on each side of your midriff, are the right and left midriff cavities. These cavities are directly connected to your middle dantian. And above them, located just below your shoulders, are the right and left armpit cavities. These two cavities are directly connected to your upper dantian (see figure 2: Taoist Subtle Anatomy, page 14). Although there are additional organs of the subtle energy field described by both Taoist and Yogic adepts—including chakras, minor energy centers, meridians, etc.—in this exercise, we would like you to focus on the dantians and smaller cavities that support them.

Exercise: A Journey through Your Subtle Field

To begin the journey through your non-physical field, find a comfortable position with your back straight. Then close your eyes and breathe deeply through your nose for two to three minutes. When you're ready to continue, go to your personal healing space and bring your awareness to your body, soul, and spirit. Enjoy your healing space for five minutes. Then assert, *"It's my intent to visualize a white screen eight feet* (two and a half meters) *in front of me."* Once the visual screen has materialized, assert, *"It's my intent to visualize an image of myself on the screen."* Keep your appropriate organs of perception (sight, hearing, feeling, and intuition) open and active because it's by turning the appropriate organs of perception inward, on the subtle planes, that you will perceive the organs of your subtle field. Your organs of perception include your senses (which gather physical-material input) as well as your other, non-physical means of knowing, such as intuition.

After you've examined your image from eight feet (two and a half meters) away, assert, *"It's my intent to visualize the organs of my subtle field described by the Taoists."* Immediately, the physical image will give way to an image that appears almost transparent. As soon as you view the transparent image, assert, *"It's my intent to project myself inside my subtle field alongside my lower dantian."* Use all the appropriate senses to examine the lower dantian. Reach out and touch it. Feel the pressure and texture of its surface boundary. Pay attention to everything you see and feel. Even your emotional state and your body awareness can provide you with valuable information. If you suddenly feel weak or stressed, or you feel pressure and/or mild pain for no apparent reason, it could mean that the dantian contains distorted energy.

Don't be concerned if, at first, you experience a featureless cavity in the center of your abdomen. If you're centered in your subtle field and remain patient, features will begin to emerge. You may notice that the surface boundary is composed of luminous fibers that crisscross each other in every direction. You may also notice that the surface boundary is not uniform and that some of the energy in the dantian is heavier and darker and more active than the background energy within it. The background energy is chi. Since chi only has universal qualities, it will always appear clear and light—and it will always have a uniform quality. On the other hand, distorted energy has individual qualities such as color, weight, density, and level of activity. The heavier, darker, and more active the energy appears to be, the more distorted and disruptive it will be.

After you've observed the lower dantian for one to two minutes, assert, *"It's my intent to project myself alongside my middle dantian and to observe its features."* Take one to two minutes to observe the condition of your middle dantian. Then assert, *"It's my intent to project myself alongside my upper dantian and observe its features clearly."* Follow the same routine with the upper dantian that you did with the lower two dantians. Then assert, *"It's my intent to project myself beside my left kwa."* Observe its condition for one to two minutes. Then continue in the same way with your right kwa, left midriff cavity, right midriff cavity, left armpit cavity, and finally your right armpit cavity.

When you're satisfied with what you've learned, assert, *"It's my intent to return to my original position eight feet in front of my visual screen."* Release the image of yourself and the visual screen next. Then assert, *"It's my intent to leave my healing space."* Continue by counting

from one to five. When you reach the number five, open your eyes—
and bring yourself out of the exercise.

After you've taken your first journey through your subtle field, you can refine
your ability through repetition. Even if you had only limited success, with
practice, your ability will improve—and in time, you will be able to use all of
your organs of perception as well as your intent and mental attention to experience the organs and systems that compose your subtle field.

Petra continued to perform the journey through her subtle field for several weeks. Later, she got permission from her partner to perform a journey
through his subtle field. (It's essential to get permission before you enter another person's field of energy and consciousness). And it wasn't long before
her discernment improved to the point that she was able to observe many
additional features of the subtle energy field, including chakras, meridians,
and minor energy centers.

After Petra was able to use her enhanced discernment to observe the condition of Sarah's dantians, we taught her to release blockages and replace them
with life-affirming prana and to overcome trauma scars, which you will learn
to do later in this book. Due to her efforts, it didn't take her long to heal Sarah's
sleep problem as well as to enhance her vitality and reduce her anxiety.

— TWO —
Take Control of Your Subtle Field

The consciousness (vijnana) and energy (prana) that compose your subtle field both have universal qualities, which means that they are life-affirming and they support family relationships. Examples of life-affirming qualities include respect for women and children as well as discipline, courage, patience, perseverance, loyalty, long-suffering, and non-harming. It's qualities such as these that allow a family member to express themselves as they truly are, without the burden of attachments and negative patterns getting in the way. And it's qualities such as these that indicate that a family member has the space within their subtle field to empathize with the people they love.

If consciousness and energy with universal qualities were all that existed and the authentic mind was the only vehicle of awareness in the physical and non-physical universe, then all human relationships would be joyful and satisfying. But relationship problems with family members plague most people's lives—which means that alongside energy and consciousness with universal qualities there must be (another form of) energy and consciousness that support patterns, attachments, and even obsessions—all of which can disrupt well-being and intimate, long-term relationships.

Energy and Consciousness with Individual Qualities
Other forms of subtle energy and consciousness do exist. They have individual qualities and they can change form, texture, and level of activity without warning. We've worked with them on countless occasions because, in almost

all cases, they support the divisive relationship issues that pull family members apart.

Energy with individual qualities is easy to recognize because it feels dense and heavy. And it creates pressure and muscle-ache as well as anxiety, depression, self-doubt, and confusion when it interacts with your subtle field. Unlike prana (chi), it moves in waves that have what you can think of as character—or what we call a "flavor." In most cases, the flavor is unpleasant because energy with individual qualities, when present in your subtle field, will block the flow of prana radiating through it. And it's prana which serves as the foundation of all universal qualities including pleasure, love, intimacy, and joy.

Consciousness with individual qualities can burst or slowly blanket your awareness with attitudes and ideas that create confusion. It can also create self-doubt and obsessive thoughts that can compel you to act in hurtful ways or to hold on to beliefs that have their foundation in self-limiting fields of consciousness.

If enough fields of energy and consciousness with individual qualities become trapped in your subtle field and you become attached to them because you believe they are "real" (generated by your authentic mind), you can create an inauthentic mind which will function in opposition to your authentic mind. This mind has two parts, the "I," which creates a false identity, and the ego, which manifests a false personality. Together they can disrupt your ability to be yourself, express yourself freely, and engage in life-affirming family relationships.

Although the individual mind and ego are self-serving and often narcissistic, they can be restrained so that they serve rather than interfere with your relationships. This is a goal of both Yoga and Taoism as well as deep family healing.

The ability to restrain the individual mind and ego is not something reserved for Yogic adepts or enlightened prophets. It's something anyone with the yearning to be free and to be themselves can do.

Our continuing work with Andrew and his family illustrates how the individual mind and ego can interfere with your family relationships and how, with knowledge and skill, they can be made to serve you so that the process of deep family healing can proceed without disruption.

You were introduced to Andrew in the introduction to this book. In his first session with us, we learned that his father, Frank, had been a violent man whose words and actions had created a climate of fear in the family. Frank eventually abandoned Andrew and his mother when Andrew was six years old. To compensate for his feelings of pain and loss—as well as the pervasive anxiety he experienced—Andrew attached himself to subtle fields of energy and consciousness with individual qualities, which his father had projected into his subtle field. These fields, although not part of his authentic mind or subtle field, provided him with two things he desperately needed at the time—the feeling and belief that he was in control of his life. Unfortunately, these same projections compelled him to put his own needs first in virtually every interaction with other people, including his children—just like his father had done.

Although Andrew wanted nothing to do with his father, it was clear to us that he was still deeply attached to him. That's because Andrew's attachment to his father's projections bound him to his father on the subtle levels of energy and consciousness. In addition, the core values he embraced compelled him to put personal survival above the needs of his wife and children.

We recognized early in our work with Andrew that the process required to heal the family dynamic would span three generations. This meant that to understand and participate fully in the process, Andrew needed to know how fields of consciousness and energy with individual qualities projected by his parents disrupted his development and his relationship to his wives and children.

Development of the Individual Mind and Ego

After Andrew had succeeded in creating his personal healing space, we explained that there are distinct stages in the development of the individual mind and ego, which coincide with a human being's physical growth and sexual development. Of course, it's not preordained that a child must go through all these stages. But because of the acculturation process, family attachments, and the legacy of past life karma, most children do.

In the first stage, which begins at birth and lasts about seven years, a child normally remains centered in their authentic mind, and the individual mind and ego rarely have the power to disrupt their experience of intimacy. This was not the case with Andrew's son, who suffered a birth trauma during delivery. He was a large baby and got stuck in the birth canal. As a result, the delivery had to be completed using suction.

As a child grows older, however, there will be a shift of attention towards the external world that coincides with greater identification with the individual mind and ego. It's during the second stage, between the ages of seven and twelve, that many children become aware of the legacy of past action and the limitations imposed on them and their free range of activities by karmic baggage.

Karmic baggage is the accumulated amount of energy and consciousness with individual qualities that a person carries in their subtle field from one lifetime to another. As attachment grows during the third and fourth stage of personality development, between the ages of thirteen and early adulthood, the growing child will begin to experience a more fixed personality and rigid orientation towards themselves and the external world. It's during these stages, at least for some children, that the individual mind and ego eclipse the functions of the authentic mind and become dominant.

Attachment to the individual mind and ego brings with it an end to unlimited access to the authentic mind, which was a hallmark of childhood. This loss has far-reaching consequences since access to the authentic mind and the pleasure, love, intimacy, and joy that emerge from it will determine whether an adult will be able to successfully engage in long-term, intimate relationships.[3]

One thing that hadn't been diminished by Andrew's difficult childhood was his curiosity. And during our explanation, Andrew peppered us with questions about the condition of his father's subtle field and how it had influenced him. We explained that his father's subtle field had been disrupted in the first stage of development (when he was about two years old), which meant he had been unable to establish an authentic identity or even feel himself clearly. His inability to feel himself indicated that he had insufficient space in his subtle field for authentic feelings and emotions to emerge and to be resolved. It also meant that he hadn't been able to develop the patience, understanding, or the empathy he needed for successful parenting.

The Anatomy of Your Subtle Field

We continued by explaining that to overcome the legacy of his past life karma and the attachments he'd inadvertently created by embracing his father's projections, Andrew needed to know that the subtle field contains two types of energetic vehicles. Both vehicles play an important role in energetic interactions between people in relationship.

There are energy bodies that are the same size and shape as the physical-material body. Energy bodies help a person remain stable and centered in their authentic mind. People also have sheaths that are slightly larger than energy bodies. They help people express themselves freely. And they facilitate interpersonal interactions on the physical and non-physical levels.

In addition to energetic vehicles, the subtle field contains resource fields. Resource fields provide the energy that nourish energy bodies and sheaths as well as chakras and chakra fields, meridians, auras, and minor energy centers scattered throughout the subtle field. They also nourish dantians and the neighboring cavities described by the Taoists.

Everyone has thirteen chakras in their body space. These include the seven traditional chakras, which emerge along the spine and in the head, two etheric chakras, two physical chakras, and two physical-material chakras (see figure 3: The Chakras in Body Space, page 28).

The activities performed by the chakras, particularly the thirteen chakras in body space, are especially important to the health of family relationships. They include many interactions that people mistakenly believe take place exclusively on the physical-material plane. The sense of belonging and trust, as well as the ability to express feelings and emotions freely, are examples of energetic interactions regulated by the chakras; so is the ability to share pleasure, love, and intimacy with other people. The chakras' role in these interactions points to the fact that they play a central role in maintaining the health of family relationships.

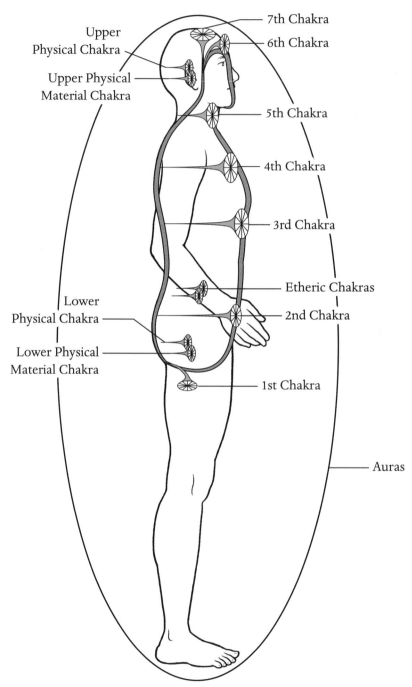

Figure 3: The Chakras in Body Space

The Chakras

The word chakra comes from Sanskrit, the sacred language of India, and means wheel. There are two distinct parts of a chakra—the chakra gate and the chakra field. For people with the ability to see non-physical energy fields, a chakra gate will look like a brightly colored disk that spins rapidly at the end of what looks like a long axle or stalk (see figure 4: The Chakra Gate, below). The wheel portion of the chakra gate is about three inches (ten centimeters) in diameter and perpetually moves or spins around a central axis. Emerging from the center of the disk are what appear to be spokes.

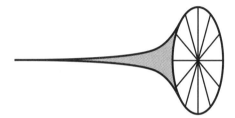

Figure 4: The Chakra Gate

Although chakra gates usually get the most attention from practitioners, the principal part of a chakra is the vast reservoir of prana and jing connected to the chakra gate, which we call the chakra field. Jing is the essence of prana (chi). You will learn how jing influences your relationships and how it can be used to heal family relationships later in this book.

In most cases, your chakra field will extend a significant distance from the surface of your physical-material body. That's because a healthy chakra field will contain a greater amount of prana and jing than a chakra field that is unhealthy. A healthy chakra field will also allow more prana and jing from the chakra field to be distributed by the chakra gate to your subtle field and physical-material body. This means that the most satisfying parts of family life—like the fullness of joy you experience watching your children play—and the amount of energy you can share with your loved ones depends primarily on the health of your chakra fields.

Chakra gates and their fields are able to perform several important functions besides providing your subtle field and physical-material body with prana and jing. They link all human beings to Universal Consciousness, the singularity from which everything in the physical and non-physical universe emerged. And they balance the forces of polarity and gender within you by permitting prana and jing to move through your subtle field in four general directions, up the back, down the front, forward from the back to the front, and backward from the front to the back.

Maintaining a healthy balance between the forces of polarity and gender will do three additional things that support family relationships. They will enhance the amount of space you have within you; they will enhance your flexibility; and they will enhance your ability to have fun, which should not be underestimated when evaluating your quality of life.

The Thirteen Chakras in Body Space

There are 146 chakras within your non-physical field. Sixty-three emerge above the top of your head and seventy emerge below your perineum. The thirteen most important chakras emerge within your body space. The thirteen chakras within body space include the seven traditional chakras that emerge along the spine and in the head, two etheric chakras, two physical chakras, and two physical-material chakras. In the following text, you will find a short list of activities regulated by these thirteen chakras.

The First Chakra emerges from the base of your spine. It regulates authentic power, security, self-confidence, body image, and your connection to the earth and its creatures. If the chakra is functioning healthfully, you will feel secure in your body and have a positive body image. You will also have a healthy relationship to the earth and its creatures.

The Second Chakra emerges four finger widths below your navel. It regulates vitality, gender identity (masculinity or femininity), creativity, and sexual love. When the chakra is functioning healthfully, your gender identity will be in balance, which means you will be able to give and receive universal masculine and feminine energy freely. And you will have access to all your creativity and personal power.

The Third Chakra emerges from your solar plexus. It regulates the energy associated with satisfaction, contentment, trust, belonging, intimacy, friendship, status, and psychic well-being. If the chakra is functioning healthfully, you will experience all the benefits that derive from your friendships, family relationships, and group affiliations.

The Fourth Chakra emerges from the center of your breastbone. It regulates self-awareness and personal rights including the right to control your physical-material body, to express your emotions, and to follow your personal dharma (life path). When the chakra is functioning healthfully, you will be self-confident and able to share your emotions and ideas spontaneously with other people.

The Fifth Chakra emerges from your neck. It regulates self-expression, unconditional joy, perseverance, and personal integrity. When the chakra is functioning healthfully, you will be able to express yourself freely, and your dominant feeling will be joy.

The Sixth Chakra emerges from your brow. It's sometimes called the third eye. It regulates personal will, awareness, memory, intuition, reasoning, and rational, deductive thought. When the chakra is functioning healthfully, you will have unrestricted awareness of both your physical-material and non-physical environments.

The Seventh Chakra emerges from your head. It provides you with access to transcendental consciousness, self-knowledge, and transcendent relationship. When it's functioning healthfully, you will recognize your dharma (life purpose) and have unrestricted access to Universal Consciousness.

The Etheric Chakras emerge from either side of your lower abdomen. They regulate authentic feelings. There are hundreds of authentic feelings that they regulate, including comfort, satisfaction, fatigue, and enthusiasm. If the chakras are functioning healthfully, you will be able to share your feelings freely—and you will enjoy an unrestricted flow of prana and jing on the etheric level.

The Physical Chakras: your upper physical chakra emerges from a position just below and behind your sixth chakra. Your lower physical chakra emerges from a position just below and in front of your second chakra. The physical chakras are responsible for regulating physical sensation and pleasure, particularly sexual pleasure.

The Physical-Material Chakras: your upper physical-material chakra emerges from a position just below your chin. Your lower physical-material chakra emerges from a position a palm's width below your perineum. The physical-material chakras are responsible for grounding you in the physical-material world. Being grounded allows you to experience your physical-material body and its environment without disruption. It also enhances your experience of union with the earth and its creatures. For the position of the thirteen chakras in body space, see figure 3: The Chakras in Body Space, page 28.

EXERCISE: Feeling the Chakras in Body Space

To facilitate Andrew's healing process—and to make him more aware of his relationship to subtle energy—we had him perform the next series of exercises. That's because even though many people have learned something about the structure and function of the chakras, they often have difficulty sensing them. This is unfortunate because prana radiating through the chakras can be used to heal many of the conditions and ailments that interfere with family relationships.

A simple way to sense the chakras is to use the power of running water to stimulate them. This is easy to do in the shower. Simply direct the stream of water from the shower head to the front of your first chakra gate, which extends from the base of your spine to a point three inches (ten centimeters) below it. Continue until you feel a vibration emerging from the point where the chakra gate is located. Take a few moments to enjoy the resonance—then move the shower head to the second chakra gate, four finger widths below your navel. After a few moments, you will feel the unique vibration of the second chakra. Continue to use the water emerging from the shower head to stimulate your third through seventh chakras, and your etheric, physical, and physical-material chakras.[4] You can see the position of the chakras by consulting figure 3: The Chakras in Body Space, page 28.

Once you're finished stimulating your chakras, take about ten minutes to enjoy their enhanced resonance, which will continue—even after you've finished stimulating them.

EXERCISE: Sensing the Chakras
in Body Space

Another way to sense the chakras in your body space is to rub your palms together and then place the palm of your "positive" hand—right if you're right-handed, left if you're left-handed—about three inches (ten centimeters) in front of each chakra gate.

Rubbing your palms together polarizes them slightly, making it easier for you to sense the resonance of each chakra consciously. If you begin by rubbing your hands together and then place your positive hand above your first chakra gate, you will activate the chakra and your palm will register its unique resonance by vibrating or glowing within the chakra's spectrum of energy.

To continue the process, simply remove your hand and rub your palms together again. Then place the palm of your positive hand in front of the second chakra gate, four finger widths below your navel. Your palm will register a slightly higher resonance than your first chakra. Continue in the same way by rubbing your palms together and then experiencing the unique resonance of the third, fourth, fifth, sixth, and seventh chakras.

Once you've experienced the resonance of the seven traditional chakras, use the same technique to sense the resonance of your etheric, physical, and physical-material chakras.

After you've finished stimulating all thirteen chakras, take a few minutes to enjoy the effects that you experience on the levels of body, soul, and spirit.

EXERCISE: Activating a Chakra

Once you can sense the resonance of your chakras in body space, you can use your intent and mental attention to activate them. In the exercise that follows, you will activate your heart chakra. The same technique can be used to activate any of your 146 chakras. Being able to activate your chakras is an essential part of many of the advanced healing techniques you will perform in deep family healing. So we recommend that you perform the exercise as part of your daily regimen of energy work.

To begin the exercise, find a comfortable position with your back straight. Then close your eyes and breathe deeply through your nose for two to three minutes. When you're ready to continue, go to your personal healing space and bring your awareness to your body, soul, and spirit. Enjoy your healing space for five minutes. Then assert in a normal voice, *"It's my intent to activate my heart chakra."* Once you've activated your heart chakra, you'll feel a growing feeling of lightness, which is accompanied by a heightened sense of well-being. You can enhance these effects by asserting, *"It's my intent to turn my appropriate organs of perception inward on the level of my heart chakra."*

By turning the appropriate organs of perception (sight, hearing, and feeling) inward, you'll become even more conscious of the shift that has taken place once you've activated your heart chakra.

Enjoy the meditation for fifteen minutes. During that time, resist the urge to drift or to follow the movement of energetic waves and/or fields. Only fields of energy with individual qualities move in waves and/or fields. And if you allow yourself to be distracted by the movement of energy with individual qualities, your chakra will become less active. After fifteen minutes, return to normal consciousness by counting from one to five. When you reach the number five, open your eyes and bring yourself out of the meditation.

Once Andrew learned to activate his chakras in body space, we taught him to enhance his discernment by taking a more comprehensive journey through his subtle field. We recommend that you take the same journey in order to familiarize yourself with the thirteen chakras in body space—and to develop your discernment.

Discernment is a form of subtle intuition that will enable you to recognize the differences between energy with universal qualities, which is the foundation of pleasure, joy, and generosity, and energy with individual qualities, which is the foundation of self-limiting qualities such as jealousy, dependency, and arrogance. By developing your discernment, you will find it easier to remain centered in energetic fields that are authentic. And in a short time, you will be able to wrest control of your subtle field back, on the energy level, from fields of energy with individual qualities.

Andrew performed the journey of discernment for several weeks because of his inability to discern the difference between fields of energy with universal qualities and fields of energy with individual qualities. The exercise turned out to be a boon for him and will be a boon for anyone who has difficulty sensing their subtle energy field and the subtle energetic interactions that take place within it.

In your journey, you will observe your chakras in body space and the fields of distorted energy that have been interfering with their ability to function healthfully. These fields will be easy to discern because they feel heavy and move in waves. And they have individual qualities such as size, shape, density, level of activity, and color. These individual qualities will stand out against the background of prana which has only universal qualities and which is light and clear and doesn't move in waves.

EXERCISE: A Journey of Discernment

To begin your journey of discernment, find a comfortable position with your back straight. Then close your eyes and breathe deeply through your nose for two to three minutes. Go to your personal healing space next and bring your awareness to your body, soul, and spirit. When you're ready to continue, assert, *"It's my intent to visualize a white screen eight feet* (two and a half meters) *in front of me."* Once the visual screen has materialized, assert, *"It's my intent to visualize an image of myself on the screen."* Keep your appropriate organs of perception (sight, hearing, feeling, intuition, etc.) open and active because it's by turning the appropriate organs of perception inward, on the subtle planes, that you will perceive the organs of your subtle field.

After you've examined your image from eight feet (two and a half meters) away, assert, *"It's my intent to visualize the organs of my subtle field described by Yogic adepts."* Immediately, the physical image will give way to an image that appears almost transparent. As soon as you view the transparent image, assert, *"It's my intent to project myself inside my subtle field alongside my first chakra."* Use all the appropriate senses to examine your first chakra gate and then the chakra field. Reach out and touch them both. Feel the pressure and texture of the surface boundary that surrounds the chakra field. Pay attention to everything you see and feel. Even your emotional state and your body awareness can provide you with valuable information. If you suddenly feel weak or stressed or you feel pressure and/or mild pain for no apparent reason, it could mean that the first chakra gate or field contains distorted energy.

After you've observed your first chakra for one to two minutes, assert, *"It's my intent to project myself alongside my second chakra and to observe its features."* Take one to two minutes to observe the condition of your second chakra. Then assert, *"It's my intent to project myself alongside my third chakra."* Continue in the same way until you've observed the seven traditional chakras along your spine and head as well as your etheric, physical, and physical-material chakras. Then assert, *"It's my intent to experience fields of distorted energy that interfere with the functions of my seven traditional chakras in body space."* Don't interact with these distorted fields; just observe them. They will stand out from the background of prana (chi), which is clear, doesn't move, and has no individual qualities.

When you're satisfied with what you've learned, assert, *"It's my intent to return to my original position eight feet in front of my visual screen."* Release the image of yourself and the visual screen next. Then assert, *"It's my intent to leave my healing space."* After you've brought yourself out of your healing space, count from one to five. When you reach the number five, open your eyes—and bring yourself out of the exercise.

———————

Andrew continued to perform the exercise regularly until he was confident that he could discern the differences between prana (chi) and energy with individual qualities. In a subsequent session, he confessed that the last thing he ever wanted was to become like his father. We understood his concern which was why we continued his healing process by helping him to restore his relationship to his parents.

At the time, Andrew still believed that his relationship issues were caused almost exclusively by his father's actions. We recognized that this was only part of the problem and that his mother, Patricia, also had an impact on his subtle field. This came as no surprise since both parents, regardless of their condition, influence the family dynamic. In Andrew's birth family, Patricia and her energetic projections contributed to the difficulty he had establishing an independent identity and healthy relationships with his wives and children.

During a subsequent session, we explained that even though his father had projected distorted energy at Andrew—in the form of cords and controlling waves—in an effort to push him away, his projections had the opposite effect. They had bound them together. That's because projections designed to push people away can cause attachments that bind people together for years or, in some cases, lifetimes.

In contrast, Patricia had projected at him in order to enhance his security and make him feel safe in what she felt was a conflict-ridden home environment. Although these projections were less intense, they were laced with worry, anxiety, and need, which had their foundation in fields of energy with individual qualities. As a result, they contributed to the problem he had developing healthy relationships to other people.

In the process of healing his family dynamic, we taught Andrew to release his attachments to both his mother and father, which he did over a period of several months.

We also recommended that he include Patricia in the healing process. There was some resistance at first on her part. But after Andrew assured her that he wanted to restore their relationship, she agreed. We met her two weeks after Andrew told her about deep family healing. During our first session with her, we explained that she and Andrew could restore their relationship by sharing life-affirming energy with one another. Once she agreed to continue, we taught Andrew and Patricia to share prana with one another from their seven traditional chakras in body space.

Like Andrew and Patricia, you can use the following exercise to enhance your relationship to a family member. It doesn't matter if the family member has initiated the rift or if they have harmed you in thought or deed. By sharing prana with them, you will enhance your ability to communicate with them in a positive and joyful way.

EXERCISE: Sharing Prana

You can perform the following exercise when you are physically next to a family member or by video-conferencing with them. To enhance the life-affirming energy that you can share with a family member when you are physically together, sit six feet apart facing them. To do the same via video conferencing, sit in front of your computer so that your body from your thighs to your head is visible in the screen. Then, along with your exercise partner, follow the following instructions. Breathe deeply through your nose for two to three minutes. Then assert, *"It's my intent to go to my personal healing space."* Once you've experienced your personal healing space, bring your awareness to your body, soul, and spirit. Enjoy the process for five minutes. Then assert, *"It's my intent to bring my mental attention to my first chakra at the base of my spine."* Take a minute or two to enjoy the glow as your chakra becomes active. Then assert along with your exercise partner, *"It's my intent to radiate prana to…* (name of your exercise partner) *from my first chakra."* Take two to three minutes to enjoy the process. Then continue in the same way with your second, third, fourth, fifth, sixth, and seventh chakras. After you've shared prana with your exercise partner from each of your seven traditional chakras, enjoy the effects for another five minutes. Then you and your exercise partner should bring yourselves out of the exercise by counting from one to five. When you reach the number five, you can both open your eyes and give each other feedback or even a hug if it feels appropriate. By repeating this exercise, you can enhance your relationship by continuing to share prana with one another.

Once Andrew had released his attachments to his father and begun to share prana with his mother, we suggested that he contact his children, which he did several weeks later. Like Patricia, his children were at first reluctant to engage in the process of deep family healing. But after they spoke with us, they finally agreed to meet Andrew and give it a try.

To heal his relationship to his children, Andrew had to overcome issues that had their foundation in incompatibility and the intrusion of distorted fields into his and his children's fields of subtle energy and consciousness. In the following chapters, you will learn how the issues of compatibility—which is determined by soul vibration, core values, and the elements—and the intrusion of distorted fields influence your relationships. Then, like Andrew and his children, you will learn how you can enhance compatibility and restore family relationships.

PART 2

Everything You Need to Know About Compatibility

In *Anna Karenina*, Leo Tolstoy wrote, "All happy families resemble one another; each unhappy family is unhappy in its own way."

Happiness and unhappiness are hard to define, and family members can experience periods of both happiness and unhappiness. In many cases, the cause of long periods of unhappiness—which can separate family members from one another—has its root in incompatibility.

In part 2 of this book, we will delve into the issue of compatibility in detail, for two reasons. The first reason is that having a compatible relationship will ensure that you and your partner will be able to work out your karmic differences amicably so that you can avoid the growth of resentment and regret. The second is that in many families, compatibility must be enhanced in order to heal the family dynamic.

— THREE —
Finding a Compatible Life Partner

In this chapter, you will learn how the issue of compatibility can influence your family relationships. After that, you will learn to determine if a potential life partner will be naturally compatible with you.

For singles, choosing a partner who is naturally compatible is an important milestone. But it's vital to recognize that compatibility is not the same as romantic love, sexual attraction—or even intimacy. All three are important elements of partnership, but while romantic love and sexual attraction can wax and wane—and intimacy can be intermittent—natural compatibility is the foundation for the vast majority of successful, long-term, intimate relationships. There are two reasons for this. The first is that natural compatibility rarely changes over time—which means partners who are naturally compatible rarely drift apart. The second reason is that natural compatibility will ensure that life partners are able to share energy and consciousness with universal qualities freely with one another. That in turn will keep these relationships in balance and guarantee that love, communication, and satisfaction have fertile ground to grow and prosper.

The issue of compatibility is also central to other family relationships, including the relationship parents and children have to each other and the relationship a grown child will have to their birth family and in-laws. In patchwork and non-traditional relationships, the issue of compatibility can extend even further to include half-brothers and half-sisters as well as adults who have close relationships with ex-partners.

In 2008, we began working with Wendy and Charlie. In their first session with us, they explained that, when they met each other, they felt like they had arrived—and that they knew that their search for a satisfying life partner was over. This was a strong indication that they were compatible life partners and that they shared the same soul vibration. Problems only emerged at home when their first child, Tim, was two and a half years old. The problem with Tim emerged gradually. However, by the time he was three, he no longer allowed his parents to cuddle with him and he screamed much of the time, except when his grandmother, who lived a short distance away, looked after him. At those times, he acted like a loving, affectionate kid and gave and received affection freely. This dynamic led us to suspect that the root of the problem was a lack of compatibility between Tim and his parents. (Please consult a medical professional if you notice dramatic physical or behavioral changes in your child.)

We began to treat the problem by explaining to Wendy and Charlie that they shared the same soul vibration. Tim, on the other hand, was the odd man out. He loved his parents—because all children do—but he didn't share the same soul vibration with them, which on a visceral level made him feel that he wasn't accepted by them—and that he'd been abandoned.

In contrast, Tim felt that his grandmother accepted him and that he belonged with her because she shared the same soul vibration with him.

Natural Compatibility

To reassure Wendy and Charlie, we explained that compatibility could be enhanced by using the techniques of deep family healing. Once we had reassured Wendy and Charlie, we went on to explain that natural compatibility must be understood in two ways—what it is and what it does. At its core, natural compatibility is a field of energy and consciousness that unites people. It does that by creating a subtle environment that enhances security, trust, belonging, understanding, and communication—all of which are associated with the third chakra. We went on to explain that family members in compatible relationships contribute to the field and draw sustenance from it, which means that it will continue to support them throughout their journey on earth. Since people who are naturally compatible feel familiar and feel like they belong with one another, it mitigates against feelings of loneliness, abandonment, and separation.

In the following pages, we will look at the essential elements of natural compatibility, which include soul vibration, core values, and dominant elements. Before we do that, however, it's important to remember that although natural compatibility is the ideal, not all people in family relationships are naturally compatible in all three areas. That's why we want to stress once again that compatibility can be enhanced in any area where it's lacking— which means that family members who make the effort to enhance their compatibility with one another will be handsomely rewarded with almost all the benefits of natural compatibility. We will begin our examination of compatibility by looking at soul vibration.

Compatibility and Soul Vibration

While it's true that all human beings have a soul that includes intellect, rational, and intuitive mind as well as authentic emotions and feelings, it doesn't mean that all people have the same soul vibration.

Soul vibration is determined by many factors, including where a person's soul originated (not all souls originated on earth), how many lives the soul has experienced, and where the soul has lived during this life and its previous incarnations—as well as a person's activities and experiences in past incarnations, especially those that were violent and left energetic wounds and trauma scars in their subtle field (for more on energetic wounds and trauma scars, go to chapter 12).

The combination of factors mentioned above explains why not all souls in their current condition are naturally compatible with one another or capable of experiencing all the pleasure, love, intimacy, and joy available to them. It also explains why elders, in many traditional societies, took the soul vibration of prospective partners seriously enough to consult astrologers and professional match-makers before a match was made. Systems of astrology in both East and West used the position of the planets at birth and their interactions to discern whether the soul vibrations of prospective partners were compatible, and match-makers used their insight and intuition to reach the same conclusion.

Compatible Soul Vibrations

When family members have compatible soul vibrations, they will feel comfortable with one another, understand one another, and they will have a strong foundation for intimacy. This will make it easy for family members to shift their orientation from Me to We. And it will make it easier for them to share pleasure, love, intimacy, and joy with one another. Family members with the same soul vibration will naturally respect each other, and they will enhance each other's best qualities. They will be able to share more activities than family members whose soul vibrations aren't naturally compatible—and they will find it easy to compromise and reconcile their differences.

In addition, family members that have compatible soul vibrations will be naturally generous to one another and will enthusiastically participate in frequent gift-giving. In fact, frequent gift-giving and other signs of affection are clear signs that partners share the same soul vibration.

Incompatible Soul Vibrations

Partners with incompatible soul vibrations will not feel like they have arrived, although they will often experience a yearning to unite as well as intense feelings of romantic love at the onset of their relationship. However, in most cases these intense feelings—particularly the intense yearning to unite—indicate a deeper problem, which is often overlooked. That is the need to overcome subtle energetic barriers to love and intimacy. These subtle barriers emerge when partners are attracted to one another, but their soul vibrations are incompatible.

Attraction can be created in many ways. It can be created by compatibility. But it can also be created by past life, karmic attachments; by cultural programming; and by attachments to distorted fields of energy and consciousness that are shared by both partners. However, attraction without compatibility can create striving, which can block the flow of prana through a person's subtle field. That in turn can enhance feelings of loneliness, which would seem out of place in a healthy relationship.

When a parent and child don't share the same soul vibration, the third chakras of both family members will be affected. As a result, the sense of belonging can be disrupted. This can make the child feel that they don't belong or that there is something wrong with them. And it can make a parent feel that there is an invisible barrier that separates them from their child. This can lead a parent to the spurious conclusion that they lack parental love or, if there is more than one child in the family, that they care for one child more than the other.

Compatibility and Core Values

Core values also influence compatibility. That's because core values represent what people believe in, have faith in, and want most. Core values also influence how a person interacts with their family members and how they view themselves in relation to the world around them.

Healthy family relationships require that family members share core values that are life-affirming. By life-affirming, we don't mean positive; with a little effort, a negative core value can be spun into something that appears positive—but is not. Thus, greed can be spun into a desire for success and prosperity. Control can be spun into the desire to make the world a better place. And dependency and neediness can be spun into caring or even romantic love.

Examples of core values that are life-affirming include generosity, empathy, playfulness, and respect for others as well as all other qualities that enhance communication and understanding.

Family members with core values that are life-affirming are always compatible because life-affirming core values will do two things: they will support the free radiation of consciousness and energy with universal qualities, and they will support a family member's purpose for being incarnated in this life.

Incompatible Core Values

When people in the same family don't share life-affirming core values, they won't have the relationship skills or energetic support they need to overcome internal and external threats to their family relationships. As a result, discord and misunderstanding will replace harmony and receptivity, and communication and understanding will be in short supply. The following examples will illustrate what we mean.

One family we worked with included a father whose name was Randy. He was old-school and believed that children should not talk during dinner and should even refrain from drinking until they had finished the meal. For Randy, a distorted form of discipline was paramount. In contrast, the children's mother, Laura, had a different set of core values. She felt that the children should enjoy themselves during dinner and express themselves freely. These opposing core values surfaced at meal times and created a divisive environment, which frightened the children and pulled their parents apart.

When their son William and daughter Lilith, who were two years apart, reached puberty, they developed difficulties which included polarity problems that interfered with their development and peer relationships. William had suffered most from the family dynamic. His father's self-limiting core values and extreme gender orientation had disrupted his up-down polarity to such an extent that he developed a condition called reversed polarity. Lilith's polarity problem was less severe, but it had also disrupted her development. In chapter 5, you will learn how William and Lilith restored their polarity to a healthy balance.

Like Randy, Andrew had become attached to a set of self-limiting core values that interfered with his family relationships. That's because Andrew's father had been violent and self-centered and had projected fields of energy with individual qualities into Andrew's subtle field. In time, these projections produced core values that justified Andrew's narcissism and self-limiting life strategy.

Compatibility and the Elements

Andrew had an additional compatibility problem. He had married his second wife in 2007. Although they shared the same soul vibration, problems soon developed because they didn't share the same core values or dominant elements.

To help Andrew and his second wife restore their elemental compatibility, we began by explaining that Chinese adepts were the first to recognize that the elements water, metal, earth, wood, and fire could influence family relationships. They discovered that a person's dominant element exerted a powerful influence on how they interacted with other people and the physical-material environment. They also learned that a person's dominant element influenced their character, particularly how disciplined, loyal, patient, and perseverant they would be—as well as whether they would be able to maintain their integrity during difficult times (long-suffering) and whether they'd refrain from harming people in word, thought, and deed.

We've found that relationship partners whose dominant elements are in harmony will experience many benefits. They will have a deep, natural affinity for one another. In most cases, the affinity will be both sexual and spiritual because the partners will be sharing the same outlook on life—which will make the relationship intoxicating for them both.

In the classical world, this natural affinity included the notion of "love at first sight," which occurs when partners first meet. According to the ancient Greeks, this phenomenon includes the projection of "love arrows" or "love darts." If these arrows arrived at the lover's eyes, they would "pierce" their heart, overwhelming them with longing, and producing *theia mania*, "madness from the gods."[5]

Incompatible Elements

When partners have dominant elements that are not compatible, then friction and misunderstanding are inevitable. It's important to note that incompatible elements can be deceptive, acting much like opposites that can attract people to one another. Unfortunately, in the long term, the intensity and passion created by incompatible elements will devolve into mistrust and resentment that will drive partners apart. That's because the striving (energetic push and pull) caused by incompatible elements can cause energetic attachments and blockages that, over time, will limit both partners' ability to radiate prana freely.

In the worst-case scenario, attachments caused by incompatible elements can disrupt empathy and create a situation in which one family member dominates the other to the detriment of them both and to other family members.

Although this process had not proceeded too far in Andrew's second marriage, both he and his wife agreed that Andrew's view of relationship had become more patriarchal and judgmental over the years. They also agreed that he had trouble listening to other people, especially when they disagreed with him.

In the next chapter, you will find out how Andrew and his second wife and son harmonized their core values and dominant elements. Before we do that, however, you will learn to determine if a prospective partner will be naturally compatible with you.

Choosing a Compatible Life Partner

For those of you who are single or who haven't committed to a long-term relationship, choosing a life partner who is naturally compatible with you can help you avoid many relationship problems that can disrupt family relationships and the condition of your subtle field.

To discern if a potential life partner is naturally compatible with you, you must begin by enhancing your inner vision. Your inner vision is a natural function of your sixth chakra, the third eye. And it's your third eye that will enhance your discernment, the ability to look into the subtle dimensions where fields of distorted energy and karmic baggage are located.

Enhancing your inner vision is a two part process. In the first part, you will learn to perform the Inner Vision Mudra. The Inner Vision Mudra was designed specifically to enhance your discernment and your ability to trust it. After you've learned to perform the Inner Vision Mudra, you will move on to the Eye of Brahma Technique. The Eye of Brahma Technique will help you to determine whether a lack of compatibility with a potential partner or a family member has interfered with the relationship.

By mastering these two exercises, you will have the skills necessary to determine whether you and a potential partner will be naturally compatible or whether incompatibility has interfered with a family relationship.

EXERCISE: The Inner Vision Mudra

To perform the Inner Vision Mudra, find a comfortable sitting position with your back straight. Breathe deeply through your nose for two to three minutes. Then put the pads of your thumbs together as far as the first joint. Twist your index fingers around each other and place the pads of the fingers together from the tip to the first joint. Then twist your middle fingers around each other so that the pads of the fingers are touching one another as far as your first joint. Your ring fingers and pinkies should be pulled into their corresponding palms. Once your hands are in position, continue by placing the tip of your tongue on your upper palate and sliding it straight back until it comes to rest at the point where the hard palate rolls up and becomes soft. Then put the soles of your feet together and close your eyes (see figure 5: The Inner Vision Mudra, page 51). Hold the mudra for ten minutes. After ten minutes, release the mudra and open your eyes.

We recommend that you practice the mudra every day for at least two weeks. After two weeks or when you're satisfied that you've received the benefits of the Inner Vision Mudra, you can begin practicing the Eye of Brahma Technique.

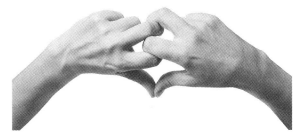

Figure 5: The Inner Vision Mudra

The Eye of Brahma

The Eye of Brahma is the inner eye. It's sometimes called the eye of wisdom. While the physical eyes see things in the material world, the Eye of Brahma sees things in the subtle world where truth can be recognized without the distortion of time and space. The Eye of Brahma should not be confused with the third eye. While the third eye is part of your subtle energy field and regulates intuition and discernment, the Eye of Brahma is part of your subtle field of consciousness. By centering yourself in the Eye of Brahma, you will be firmly rooted in the truth that you see and feel when your third eye is active.

There is a Zen story which explains how the Eye of Brahma can help you to see the truth clearly and thereby recognize an appropriate life partner. It goes like this:

There lived a monk who was new to Buddhist study and meditation. One day after a class, he approached a senior monk and asked him, "Brother! A Bodhisattva [living Buddha] has a thousand eyes; how many eyes are true?" The senior monk replied, "Only one is true." The new student doubted this and persisted by asking a further question: "Why is only one eye true, brother?" The answer he received was this: "The one true eye is the wisdom that is within each person. Let us consider the actions of a blind man and how he reaches out for this and that without seeing. In the morning, when your alarm clock rings, you switch it off without opening your eyes. Which eye are you and the blind man using?" The new monk answered, without hesitation, "Yes, that must be the Eye of Wisdom, brother. I understand now that the Eye of Wisdom is the only one that sees the truth without the distortions of the world interfering."[6]

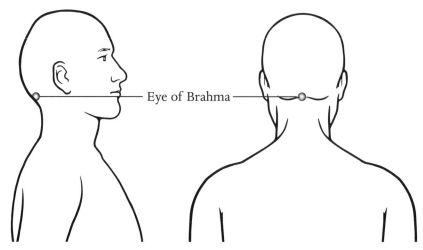

Figure 6: The Eye of Brahma

EXERCISE: The Eye of Brahma Technique

To perform the Eye of Brahma Technique, find a comfortable sitting position with your back straight. Breathe deeply through your nose for two to three minutes. Then go to your personal healing space and bring your awareness to your body, soul, and spirit. Take two to three minutes to enjoy the changes you experience. Then place your index finger at the back of your neck. Continue by sliding your index finger slowly up the center of your neck till you reach a small bump in the back of your head. That bump is located just outside the cerebellum. If you move your mental attention inward from the back of the cerebellum two inches (five centimeters), you will reach the Eye of Brahma (see figure 6: The Eye of Brahma, above). Once your mental attention reaches the Eye of Brahma, you will experience a glow emanating from that point. Enjoy the glow for another five minutes. Then release your mental attention and leave your personal healing space by asserting, *"It's my intent to return to normal consciousness."* Continue by counting from one to five. When you reach the number five, open your eyes and bring yourself out of the meditation.

We recommend that you practice the Eye of Brahma Technique until you are confident that you can enjoy the Eye of Brahma without distraction for at least five minutes.

EXERCISE: Determining Relationship Compatibility

Once you're satisfied that you can perform the Eye of Brahma Technique and the Inner Vision Mudra, you can use them to determine whether someone is naturally compatible with you and therefore an appropriate life partner. You can also use the same process to determine if a family member is compatible with you or not. Determining compatibility is a four-day process.

Day 1–3: On the first three days, find a comfortable position with your back straight before going to bed. Then perform the Inner Vision Mudra (see figure 5: The Inner Vision Mudra, page 51). Hold the mudra for five minutes with your eyes closed. Then release the mudra and go to your personal healing space. Once you've brought your awareness to your body, soul, and spirit, bring your mental attention to your Eye of Brahma and assert, *"It's my intent to center myself in the Eye of Brahma."* Continue by asserting, *"It's my intent to turn my appropriate organs of perception inward to the Eye of Brahma."* Take ten minutes to enjoy the shift. Then count from one to five. When you reach the number five, open your eyes and bring yourself out of the exercise. Then go directly to bed.

Day 4: On the fourth day, find a comfortable position with your back straight before going to bed. Then close your eyes and breathe deeply through your nose for two to three minutes. Next, perform the Inner Vision Mudra and hold it for the remainder of the exercise. To continue, assert, *"It's my intent to center myself in the Eye of Brahma."* Take a few moments to enjoy the shift. Then assert, *"It's my intent to turn my appropriate organs of perception inward on the level of the Eye of Brahma."* Stay centered in the Eye of Brahma for five minutes. Then assert, "*It's my intent to know if...* (name of the potential partner) *is an appropriate life partner for me.*" To determine if there is a lack of compatibility that disrupts your relationship with a family member, assert, "*It's my intent to know if...* (name of family member) *and I have a compatibility issue with one another.*" Stay centered for another five minutes. Then release the Inner Vision Mudra, and bring yourself out of the exercise by counting from one to five. When you reach the number five, open your eyes and go to bed. By morning—either through insight, intuition, or dreams—you will be able to discern the energetic condition of the potential life partner and/or family member. And you will know if the relationship you have in mind is appropriate. In the case of a family member, you will know whether a compatibility issue has been driving you apart.

Muscle Testing

Even though the techniques you just learned will help you discern if a potential life partner is naturally compatible with you, we've included another technique in this chapter that will validate your results. It's called muscle testing. Since committing yourself to a long-term relationship is such a major decision, we recommend that you use muscle testing after you've performed the Inner Vision Mudra and the Eye of Brahma Technique to confirm your results.

Muscle testing is used to test the body's responses when applying pressure to a large muscle. Muscle testing can be used to validate what you've learned through the Inner Vision Mudra and the Eye of Brahma Technique. And it can provide you with information about energy blockages, the condition of your organs, nutritional deficiencies, and food allergies.

Muscle testing is based on two principles. The first principle states that your body knows what is appropriate for you, even when your intellect does not. The second states that your muscle tone will get weaker when the body sends out a No response and stronger when it sends out a Yes response.

Muscle testing requires some practice (and usually is performed with a partner) in order to recognize a true Yes and No. Therefore, before you use it for important life questions like the appropriateness of a partnership, you should practice muscle testing to determine whether eating certain foods or wearing certain clothes is appropriate. All questions you propose should have a simple yes or no answer.

To avoid confusion, we recommend that you perform muscle testing on your own. To do that, you can use the Finger Ring Technique.

EXERCISE: The Finger Ring Technique

In this exercise, you will use muscle testing to confirm what you learned about your potential partner in the preceding exercise. To begin, formulate the question you want to ask. Always pose your query as a simple yes or no statement. In this exercise, your question will be: "Is it appropriate for me to engage in a long-term, intimate relationship with … (name)?" As soon as you pose your question, find a comfortable position with your back straight. You can stand or sit. Once you're comfortable, close your eyes and breathe deeply through your nose for two to three minutes. Then perform the Inner Vision Mudra (see figure 5: The Inner Vision Mudra, page 51). Hold the mudra for five minutes. Then release it and form a loop by bringing the tips of your thumb and index finger of your left hand together. Next, bring the thumb and index finger of your right hand inside the loop and form a second loop so that the four fingers look like two links of a chain. As soon as your fingers are in position, assert in a normal voice, *"It's appropriate for me to engage in a long-term intimate relationship with … (name)."* Immediately, without violence, but with all of your strength, try to pull the loops apart. If you can pull the loops apart, then it's not appropriate to engage in an intimate relationship with that particular person. You can validate your finding by making the opposite statement: "It's not appropriate for me to engage in a long-term, intimate relationship with … (name)." Then once again form two loops with your fingers and use all your strength to pull them apart. If you have performed the exercise correctly, you will find that you cannot pull them apart, and that will serve as an additional validation.

— FOUR —
Enhancing Compatibility

In this chapter you will learn to enhance soul vibration compatibility with a family member if it's lacking. Enhancing compatibility on the level of soul is not only possible but relatively easy to do. That's because everyone's subtle field shares the same structure and functions in the same way, which means that, once family members can share energy and consciousness freely, they will break down the barriers that support incompatibility.

However, before you learn to enhance compatibility on the level of soul, you must be able to sense your own soul vibration. In order for you to do that, we've developed an exercise called the Soul Vibration Mudra. We taught this technique to Wendy and Charlie, whose family problems began with the birth of their first child, Tim.

They performed the exercise together every day for several weeks. We were gratified to learn that they quickly recognized two significant things: they shared the same soul vibration, which validated our original insight; and, because they didn't share the same soul vibration with Tim, they hadn't been able to empathize with him or bond with him on the subtle levels of energy and consciousness. These two insights motivated Wendy and Charlie to use the techniques of deep family healing to restore their relationship to Tim and put their son's needs above their own.

We also taught this exercise to Andrew after we explained the principles of compatibility to him. He practiced it for several weeks before he called his ex-wife, Shelly, who had a different soul vibration. He was able to convince

Shelly to participate in the healing process by explaining that he wanted to heal his relationship to her and to his oldest son, Mark. After Mark agreed to participate, all three family members learned to perform the following series of exercises—and within a short time they were able to harmonize their soul vibrations.

EXERCISE: The Soul Vibration Mudra

To perform the Soul Vibration Mudra, find a comfortable position with your back straight. Breathe deeply through your nose for two to three minutes. Then place the tips of your thumbs together and the tips of your index fingers together. By doing that, you will create a triangle which you should hold in front of your solar plexus. Let your other fingers drop loosely towards your palms without them touching and don't do anything special with your tongue or feet (see figure 7: The Soul Vibration Mudra, page 59).

Hold the mudra for ten minutes with your eyes closed. After ten minutes, release the mudra and open your eyes. By practicing the mudra regularly, you will quickly be able to sense your own soul vibration. And as a bonus, you will recognize, like Wendy and Charlie did, that you're part of a community of people who share the same soul vibration.

Once you can sense your personal soul vibration, you can begin to harmonize it with a family member whose soul vibration differs from yours. To harmonize your soul vibrations, you will perform a series of three exercises designed specifically for that purpose. In the first exercise, which you and your exercise partner will perform alone, you will strengthen your gaze and your ability to focus it. Being able to focus your gaze without distraction is important because your eyes, along with your hands, feet, and chakras, are the primary organs through which you share prana with other people. By performing the exercise, you will be able to gaze at your partner without being distracted. And at the same time, you will be able to share prana with them through your eyes, which is an essential part of the process.

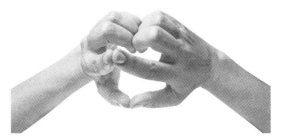

Figure 7: The Soul Vibration Mudra

EXERCISE: Strengthening Your Gaze

To strengthen your gaze, you will need a large mirror, which you will place in front of you so that you can see your face clearly. Once you've set the mirror in place, sit in front of it with your back straight. Then close your eyes and breathe deeply through your nose for two to three minutes. Go to your personal healing space next and bring your awareness to your body, soul, and spirit. Enjoy the process for five minutes. Then assert, *"It's my intent to activate my sixth chakra."* Continue by asserting, *"It's my intent to center myself in my sixth chakra field."* Take a few moments to enjoy the shift. Then assert, *"It's my intent to turn my appropriate organs of perception inward on the level of my sixth chakra field."*

Once you're centered, open your eyes (keep them slightly unfocused) and look into the eyes of your image in the mirror. Continue by asserting, *"It's my intent to radiate prana through my eyes."* Don't do anything after that. Don't try to understand what's happening or give the energy you're radiating an extra push. Just enjoy the enhanced flow of energy radiating through your eyes while you continue to make eye contact for five minutes. After five minutes, break eye contact. Then count from one to five. When you reach the number five, bring yourself out of the exercise. You and your family member should practice this exercise every day for five days or until you feel comfortable gazing and radiating prana to the image of yourselves in the mirror.

Once you and your family member feel confident that you can gaze at the image of yourself without distraction, you are ready to gaze at one another from your thirteen chakras in body space.

On the subtle levels, family members with compatible soul vibrations will share a common trait. They will be able to share prana freely from their thirteen chakra fields, in body space, while they gaze at each other. In contrast, if partners are not naturally compatible, there will be blockages which will prevent them from sharing prana in the same way.

It's important to note that each chakra regulates energetic interactions within a specific spectrum of subtle energy. If the stream of energy flowing between you and a family member, while you're centered in a chakra field, creates feelings of belonging, comfort, trust, and warmth, then you and your partner are naturally compatible within that spectrum of energy. If the stream of energy connecting you creates energetic static and angst, then you're not. You can use this principle to determine if you and your partner have compatible soul vibrations by gazing at one another while you're centered in each of your chakra fields in body space.

Gazing from the Chakras

Once you and your partner have strengthened your gaze so that you can radiate prana through your eyes without thoughts, emotions, and/or feelings interfering with it, you can begin to gaze at one another from your chakras in body space, beginning with the first chakra. After you've gazed at one another from the seven traditional chakras, you will continue with the lower and upper etheric chakras, the lower and upper physical chakras, and the lower and upper physical-material chakras (see figure 3: The Chakras in Body Space, page 28). We recommend that you gaze at one another for five minutes from each of your chakras in body space.

By gazing at one another from your chakras, you can determine whether any of the thirteen chakras in body space has been blocked and is unable to freely radiate energy and the universal qualities associated with it (see chapter 1). Blockages in the chakra fields are what create incompatibility by creating tension, stress, angst, and—in extreme cases—fear when you attempt to share prana with someone you love.

Before you begin the exercise, it's important to recognize that, when you practice mutual gazing from your chakras, you and your partner won't be staring at one another. Instead, you will be sharing universal qualities with one another while you're both centered in the appropriate chakra field.

EXERCISE: Gazing from the Chakras

To begin the exercise, find a place where you won't be distracted by other people or electronic devices. Then sit facing your partner close enough to hold hands. Keep your backs straight. Then breathe deeply through the nose for two to three minutes. Next, go to your personal healing space and bring your awareness to your body, soul, and spirit. After you've brought your awareness to your body, soul, and spirit, you can activate your first chakras by asserting, *"It's my intent to activate my first chakra."* Once the chakra is active, assert, *"It's my intent to center myself in my first chakra field."* Continue by asserting, *"It's my intent to turn my appropriate organs of perception inward on the level of my first chakra field."*

Take two to three minutes to enjoy the shift. Then begin to gaze into your partner's eyes. Don't do anything after that. Don't watch yourselves or give the prana and jing (essence) you're radiating an extra push. Just pay attention to how you feel—and whether you're able to share the universal qualities of energy associated with the chakra with your exercise partner.

After a few moments, take each other's hands so that the minor energy centers in your palms are touching. You and your exercise partner have a minor energy center in each hand that complements the functions of the chakras and enhances your ability to express yourselves and participate in worldly activities (see figure 8: Minor Energy Centers in the Hands and Feet, page 62).

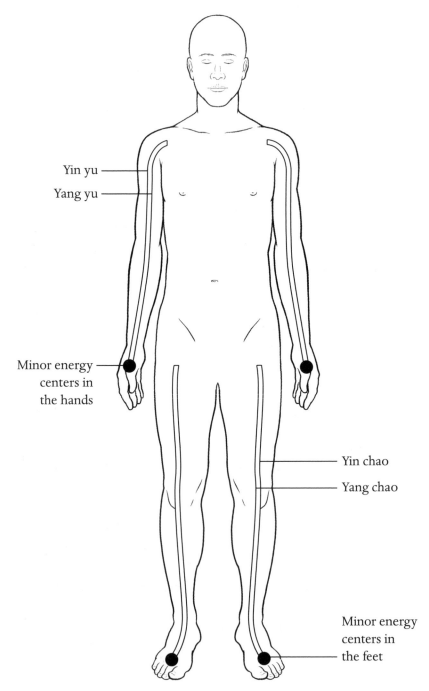

Figure 8: Minor Energy Centers in the Hands and Feet

If you and your partner can radiate prana and jing freely on the first dimension, the level of your first chakra, your breathing will get deeper and your muscles will relax. Thoughts will give way to a deep sense of well-being that will bring you closer to one another. Continue to gaze at one another for five minutes. Then release eye contact and count from one to five. When you reach the number five, bring yourselves out of the exercise. You can perform the same exercise to determine if incompatibility exists on any of the remaining dimensions, regulated by the chakras in body space.

We included a list of universal qualities associated with the thirteen chakras in body space in chapter 2. Use the list of qualities as a guide—along with feelings of static and angst and the inability to experience intimacy—to determine if compatibility has been blocked in any of your chakra fields.

Wendy and Charlie performed the exercise over a period of three weeks to determine if any of their chakras in body space were blocked. It wasn't necessary to have Tim to participate because it's quite unusual for a three-year-old to have chakras in body space that can't radiate prana and jing freely.

Both Wendy and Charlie discovered that they had blockages in their first and third chakras because of a build-up of karmic baggage as well as energetic attachments to their parents. These blockages were not strong enough to prevent them from sharing some joy with one another or from feeling like they belonged together. But they did diminish how much joy they could share and how much they could benefit from having compatible soul vibrations. That's because the first chakra plays an important part in grounding a person on earth, in feeling secure in their body, and in sharing pleasure with another person. The third chakra, which is its companion chakra, regulates belonging, contentment, trust, and feelings of security in all groups including families. Because Wendy and Charlie both had blockages in their first and third chakras, they were unable to freely share prana and jing from these chakras with their son, Tim. This was the basis of their compatibility problem with him, and why Tim felt so isolated from his parents.

As part of his healing process, Andrew performed the same exercise with his ex-wife Shelly, who didn't share the same soul vibration. By performing the exercise together, they learned that they both had blockages that interfered with the functions of their heart chakras. It's the heart chakra that regulates self-awareness and personal rights—including the right to control your physical-material body, to express your emotions, and to follow your personal dharma (life path). Because of the blockages and their inability to share prana and jing from their heart chakras freely, Shelly felt that her self-confidence and spontaneity were being blocked by Andrew. Although this wasn't Andrew's intent, their inability to interact on the subtle levels in a healthy way had exacerbated their marital problems. Although their marriage could not be restored, they could restore the compatibility of their soul vibrations. This in turn made it possible for them to work together to create a nourishing environment for their patchwork family.

Once you and a family member have checked for incompatibility by gazing from your chakras, you can begin the process of enhancing compatibility by performing the following exercise.

EXERCISE: Technique to Restore Soul Vibration Compatibility

In the following exercise, you will choose one of your chakras in body space where blockages have disrupted compatibility. Then you will activate the chakra and center yourself in the chakra field. Once you're centered, you will use your intent to fill the chakra field with prana.

By filling the chakra field with prana, you will enhance the spectrum of energy that you can share with a family member. In time, prana will fill the chakra field to capacity and reduce the influence of any karmic baggage and blockages that remain. When that happens, blockages will have less power to interfere with your relationship. That in turn will allow you to share more intimacy, empathize more deeply, and communicate more honestly with your estranged family member.

It's not necessary for you or a family member to perform the exercise together or for a small child to perform the exercise at all. Depending on your schedules, each of you can perform the exercise whenever time permits. In the following exercise, you will begin to enhance compatibility by restoring the functions of your first chakra.

Once you feel confident that you can fill a chakra field with prana, you can restore compatibility the same way in any chakra where you've discovered compatibility is lacking.

To begin the exercise, find a comfortable position with your back straight. Breathe deeply through your nose for two to three minutes. Then go to your personal healing space. Once you've brought your awareness to your body, soul, and spirit, assert, *"It's my intent to activate my first chakra at the base of my spine."* Then assert, *"It's my intent to center myself in my first chakra field."* Continue by asserting, *"It's my intent to turn my appropriate organs of perception inward on the level of my first chakra field."* Take a few moments to enjoy the shift. Then assert, *"It's my intent to fill my first chakra field with prana."* Take fifteen minutes to enjoy the effects. Then return to normal consciousness by counting from one to five. When you reach the number five, open your eyes and bring yourself out of the exercise.

We recommend that you and your partner perform the exercise every day for two weeks—or until angst and tension have been replaced by feelings of satisfaction and well-being. Once compatibility has been enhanced on one subtle dimension regulated by a chakra, continue by performing the exercise with any other chakra that has been blocked by karmic baggage, attachments, and/or distorted fields of energy.

Harmonizing Core Values

Although many couples disagree over family issues, disagreements in themselves don't indicate that partners have incompatible core values or that their core values are self-limiting. What does indicate incompatible core values or core values that are self-limiting are blockages in family relationships that prevent family members from being themselves and sharing energy with universal qualities with one another.

In contrast to self-limiting core values, core values that are life-affirming always support family relationships because they enhance the free radiation of prana and jing between family members, and they support trust, honesty, and communication. We've included a list of life-affirming core values below. This is only a partial list, but it will give you an idea of what we mean.

Life-Affirming Core Values

1. Respect for both universal feminine and masculine energy
2. Respect for women, men, and children
3. Generosity
4. Honesty
5. Flexibility
6. Self-awareness
7. Mental clarity
8. Stability and reliability
9. Empathy for others
10. Self-confidence
11. Tolerance
12. Non-harming

In the past, it was rare for societies to fully embrace life-affirming core values such as respect for people of all genders, tolerance, and empathy for others. In fact, for centuries the dominant societies in Europe, the Middle East, and America assigned a list of core values according to gender without much concern about their relationship to universal feminine and masculine energy or their effect on family relationships. Many of these societies demanded that women should be nurturing, gentle, receptive, patient, chaste, attractive, in touch with their feelings, etc. These attributes are natural to all genders. But until recently, societies in Europe, the Middle East, and America demanded that women accept them as core values while many men, especially those in authority, were free to reject them in order to embrace another set of core values that they were taught were the sole province of men. These included competitiveness, assertiveness, ambition, rationality, toughness, aggression, etc.[7]

However, for those of you who want to enhance your compatibility, it's essential that you and your partner share life-affirming core values, even if the institutions of society still don't embrace them fully.

In our work, we've learned that, in relationships where core values are not life-affirming, one partner will inevitably dominate the other. This will lead to alienation and resentment. It will also lead to disagreements that won't be settled by compromise, but by the projection of power and—in extreme cases—physical force.

Creating New Core Values

For those of you ready to enhance the compatibility of your core values, we've provided you with two exercises designed to release self-limiting core values and to replace them with core values that are life-affirming. Since all life-affirming core values are compatible, it won't be necessary to perform these exercises with a family member. Each family member can perform the exercises alone by substituting life-affirming core values for core values that are self-limiting.

The first exercise is the Orgasmic Bliss Mudra. After you've performed the Orgasmic Bliss Mudra, you will learn to perform the Core Values Transformation Technique.

Although Randy was reluctant at first to participate in the process (remember, he was old-school), three weeks of badgering by his wife and children had the desired effect. To pacify them and heal the family dynamic, he agreed to examine his core values.

Since personal reflection wasn't one of Randy's strong points, we began by teaching him to create his personal healing space. He performed this along with his wife and children for three weeks. After that, we taught him to perform the Orgasmic Bliss Mudra and the Core Values Transformation Technique. He was stubborn—but with the effects of the two exercises and a little extra prodding by his kids, he eventually softened his world view and gave them more space to be themselves.

From his father, Andrew had learned to put his personal survival above the needs of his family. To support this survival strategy, he adapted many core values that were self-limiting and in opposition to core values that were life-affirming. After Andrew restored his relationship with his mother and he'd harmonized his soul vibration with his first wife Shelly, we taught him to perform the same two exercises as Randy. By performing them every day for two and a half months, he was able to transform his core values and his relationship to his wives and children.

Irene and Simon, whom we worked with several years later, also illustrate how a couple can enhance the compatibility of their core values. Irene was brought up in a religious family and had been programmed as a child to believe that women were the weaker sex.

Simon supported that self-limiting core value—because like her, he was brought up in a patriarchal family whose mother submitted to her husband's authority.

After the birth of their daughter Elizabeth, both Irene and Simon recognized that, for their daughter's sake, it was time to change the self-limiting core values that they continued to share with their birth families. To do that, they used the Orgasmic Bliss Mudra and the Core Values Transformation Technique to release the self-limiting core value.

Since Irene was already in her early forties and had spent her life struggling with dependency issues, it was necessary for her to overcome two subordinate core values. The first was "Men can't be trusted." The second was that "A good wife submits to the will and desires of her husband."

Under our guidance, Irene repeated the process several times in order to release all three self-limiting core values and make room for life-affirming core values to replace them. Within six weeks, the condition of her subtle field improved dramatically. Prana and jing began to flow more freely through her chakra fields and major meridians. And for the first time in years, she could feel parts of her body that had been numb or off limits.

Simon released the self-limiting core value that made him feel entitled, and, a short time later, he and Irene began to share their feelings and thoughts more easily. That in turn made it easier for them to empathize with one another and to share the responsibilities of parenting.

Like Randy and Andrew, who harmonized their core values with their wives and children, and Irene and Simon, who enhanced the depth and intimacy of their relationships, you can transform your core values by performing the next two exercises.

EXERCISE: The Orgasmic Bliss Mudra

The Orgasmic Bliss Mudra is a simple technique that will allow you to experience bliss consciously. The mudra will also empower you to be yourself (your authentic self)—making it easier for you to discard core values that aren't life-affirming and that don't support family relationships.

According to Tantric adepts, orgasmic bliss is an enduring condition, deep inside your subtle field, created through the union of consciousness (Shiva) and energy (Shakti). The merging of pure consciousness and energy with universal qualities provides you with a constant flow of healing power that can release even the deepest ailments and self-limiting patterns on the level of consciousness.

By performing the Orgasmic Bliss Mudra regularly, you can expect to experience changes in your awareness and sense of Self. At first, you will experience these changes while you hold the mudra—and often for several hours afterward. Later, these changes will become a part of your day-to-day experience.

In the first significant change, your awareness will be drawn inward until it's once more centered in your body space. Three additional shifts will take place: thoughts will cease to disturb you, and you will consciously experience the life force. The life force is not something you can feel since it emerges through consciousness. But you will recognize it because it creates a buzz that enlivens your body on the molecular level.

In the final shift, the existential problem that can eat away at you from deep inside will disappear. That's because what lies at the root of the existential problem is the inability to bring bliss into your conscious awareness.

To perform the Orgasmic Bliss Mudra, sit in a comfortable position with your back straight. Then breathe deeply through your nose for two to three minutes. Continue by placing the tip of your tongue on your upper palate and sliding it straight back until it comes to rest at the point where the hard palate rolls up and becomes soft. Once the tip of your tongue is in that position, put the bottom of your feet together so that the soles are touching. Then bring your hands in front of your solar plexus and place the inside tips of your thumbs together. Continue by bringing the outside of your index fingers together from the tips to the first joint. Next, bring the outside of your middle fingers together from the first to the second joint. The fourth and fifth fingers should be curled into your palm. Once your tongue, fingers, and feet are in position, close your eyes and breathe through your nose (see figure 9: The Orgasmic Bliss Mudra).

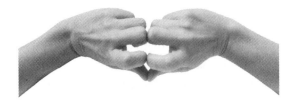

Figure 9: The Orgasmic Bliss Mudra

Hold the mudra for ten minutes. Then release your fingers, separate the soles of your feet, and bring your tongue back to its normal position.

We recommend that, like our clients, you perform the mudra every day until you feel that you've regained the clarity necessary to change negative core values into core values that are more life-affirming.

The second exercise in the process is the Core Values Transformation Technique. This exercise is designed to release self-limiting core values. Since all self-limiting core values share the same trait—they find their support in fields of distorted energy and consciousness—it's not necessary to dwell on each individual self-limiting core value. Instead, all that's necessary is to go to the place in the subtle field where core values emerge, release the distorted fields that support them, and replace them with life-affirming energy and consciousness.

The place where core values emerge and find support is known as the Core Field. It contains the sixteen functions of mind, which include intent, will, desire, resistance, surrender, acceptance, knowing, choice, commitment, rejection, faith, enjoyment, destruction, creativity, empathy, and love.

Without the support of these sixteen functions of mind, it will be difficult for a person to embrace life-affirming core values and share them with the people they love.

Before you continue, it's important to note that, when the core field is functioning healthfully, all core values will be life-affirming because the only fields that emerge from the core field will be fields of universal energy and consciousness.

EXERCISE: The Core Values Transformation Technique

When you're confident that you can experience bliss consciously, you can continue the process of transforming a core value by performing the Core Values Transformation Technique. To do that, choose a core value that you want to release. Then find a comfortable position with your back straight. Breathe deeply through your nose for two to three minutes. Then go to your healing space and bring your awareness to your body, soul, and spirit. Once you're ready to continue, perform the Orgasmic Bliss Mudra and continue to hold it throughout the exercise. After enjoying the mudra for two to three minutes, assert, *"It's my intent to center myself in my core field."* Once you're centered, assert, *"It's my intent to locate the most distorted fields of consciousness that support the core value I've chosen to release."*

Be patient because it may take a few moments for the field to emerge. As soon as it does and you recognize it by its individual qualities, you will surround it with a bliss box. To do that, assert, *"It's my intent to surround the field I observe with a bliss box."* Once the box has appeared, assert, *"It's my intent to fill the bliss box with bliss and release the distorted field of consciousness within it."* Don't do anything after that. Bliss will fill the box you've created and release the distorted field automatically.

Some of you may experience a sense of relief and/or a pop when bliss fills the box. Both indicate that the distorted field, within the bliss box, has been released and bliss has filled the empty space.

Once the distorted field has been released, release the bliss box and the Orgasmic Bliss Mudra. Then count from one to five. When you reach the number five, open your eyes. You will feel wide awake, perfectly relaxed, and better than you did before.[8]

It often takes more than one blockage to create a self-limiting core value. This means that you may have to repeat the exercise several times. Each time you repeat the exercise, release the most distorted field of consciousness. That way, you will release blockages in a systematic manner and guarantee that, in a short time, you will release the self-limiting core value you had in mind. Only then should you move on to the next self-limiting core value and release the distorted fields that support it.

EXERCISE: Filling the Core Field with Bliss

Each time you release a distorted field that supports a self-limiting core value, you can fill the core field with bliss. To do that, find a comfortable position with your back straight. Then breathe deeply through your nose for two to three minutes. Go to your healing space next and bring your awareness to your body, soul, and spirit. Once you're centered, perform the Orgasmic Bliss Mudra and hold it for the duration of the exercise. Continue by asserting, *"It's my intent to center myself in my core field."* Take a few moments to enjoy the experience. Then assert, *"It's my intent to fill my core field with bliss."* Take ten minutes to enjoy the effects physically, emotionally, and mentally. After ten minutes, release the bliss mudra and count from one to five. When you reach the number five, open your eyes and bring yourself out of the exercise.

Overcoming Elemental Incompatibility

Overcoming elemental incompatibility may seem like a hopeless endeavor. However, elemental compatibility can be enhanced by restoring the health of your domains. Everyone has three domains. They are known as the light body domain, the self-domain, and the universal domain.

It's through your three domains that the universal part of your authentic mind, *paramatman*, perceives the universe. What you may not know is that these three domains also have a significant influence on elemental compatibility because contained within them are the seeds of all five elements: water, metal, earth, wood, and fire.

Problems of elemental incompatibility are created when either the light body, Self, or universal domain have been polluted by fields of distorted energy and consciousness. Since all five elements exist within each domain, differing only in how they manifest their universal qualities, it's possible to restore elemental compatibility by restoring the functions of the domains.

However, before you can determine where incompatibility exists, you must know which qualities are manifested by each element.

Metal manifests its qualities in all three domains as self-awareness and memory. It supports the subtle field and will keep it strong and stable, even in chaotic situations. It enhances moral and physical courage, honesty, and your ability to accept your personal limitations. Normal metal enhances perseverance and supports discipline especially during times of loss and confusion.

Water manifests its qualities in all three domains as a strong sense of belonging and inner peace. It enhances emotional stability and strength and the ability to express authentic emotions at the appropriate time.

Fire is associated with the two midriff cavities as well as the universal domain. It enhances your ability to express human love and share pure consciousness. It also enhances creativity and helps motivate you to perform activities that support your dharma.

Earth is associated with being grounded in the physical-material world. It's also associated with strength in the lower dantian and kwas, both of which support the lower abdomen with chi and jing. A person with normal earth will be emotionally stable and realistic. They will find it easy to stay centered in their authentic mind, and they will have a good relationship to the earth and its creatures in all three domains.

Wood is associated with original ideas and creativity, which means it's connected to the etheric chakras and the midriff cavities. It supports motivation and the ability to make original connections that lead to advancements in the arts and sciences. Spontaneity and the acceptance of diversity are markers of a normal wood element. People with a healthy wood element are disciplined, well organized, and punctual. They play by the rules—and are trustworthy. As a result, they quickly earn the trust of their friends and colleagues. Clarity and originality are also markers of normal wood, in all three domains—so is a lifestyle that is rich in earthly benefits.

You can begin to harmonize your dominant element with a family member by performing the next exercise. We call it Gazing into Elemental Fields. It will help you to determine where elemental incompatibility exists. To do that, you must recognize that it's through the light body domain that the elements manifest their qualities as fields of universal energy. It's through the self-domain that the elements manifest their qualities as authentic identity, and it's through the universal domain that the elements manifest their qualities as paramatman, the universal Self.

In the exercise, you and your partner will center yourselves in your light body domain. Then you will gaze at one another for five minutes. If either partner experiences angst, fear, or prolonged discomfort, then you've located an area of elemental incompatibility. It's not necessary for both partners to experience discomfort for elemental incompatibility to exist.

In contrast, if you and your partner feel drawn to one another and experience a deep sense of belonging and satisfaction when you gaze at each other from the your light body domain, then you are compatible in all the universal qualities in your light body domains.

EXERCISE: Gazing into Elemental Fields

This is a partner exercise. To begin, sit one yard (meter) apart, facing one another. Once you're both comfortable, breathe deeply through your noses for two to three minutes. Then assert, *"It's my intent to center myself in my light body domain."* To continue, assert, *"It's my intent to turn my appropriate organs of perception inward on the level of my light body domain."* Take five minutes to enjoy the shift. Then open your eyes and gaze at one another for the next five minutes. Don't do anything after that. Don't watch yourself or try to enhance any of the effects. Just pay attention to whether you're able to share the universal qualities of the domain with one another. After five minutes, count from one to five and bring yourselves out of the exercise.

Once you've performed this exercise in all three domains and determined where you and your partner experience elemental incompatibility, you can use the Orgasmic Bliss Mudra along with the Bliss Box Technique to release blockages in the domains where compatibility has been disrupted. You will learn to perform the technique using the light body domain. After that, you can use the same technique to enhance compatibility in the self-domain and the universal domain.

EXERCISE: Enhancing Elemental Compatibility

To begin the exercise, find a comfortable position with your back straight. Then breathe deeply through your nose for two to three minutes. Perform the Orgasmic Bliss Mudra next (see figure 9: The Orgasmic Bliss Mudra, page 70). Continue to hold the mudra while you assert, *"It's my intent to center myself in my light body domain."* Continue by asserting, *"It's my intent to turn my appropriate organs of perception inward on the level of my light body domain."* Once you're centered, assert, *"It's my intent to surround the most disruptive blockage in my light body domain with a bliss box."* Once you can sense and/or see the box, assert, *"It's my intent to fill the box with bliss and release the disruptive blockage within it."* Don't do anything after that. Bliss will fill the box you've created and release the blockage automatically.

Some of you may experience a sense of relief and/or a pop when bliss fills the box. Both indicate that the blockage, within the bliss box, has been released and bliss has filled the empty space.

Once the blockage has been released, release the bliss box and the Orgasmic Bliss Mudra. Then count from one to five. When you reach the number five, open your eyes. You will feel wide awake, perfectly relaxed, and better than you did before.

It often takes more than one blockage to disrupt elemental incompatibility in a domain, which means that you may have to repeat the exercise in the same domain several times. Each time you repeat the exercise, release the most disruptive blockage. This way, you will release blockages in a systematic manner. We recommend that you and your partner continue to release blockages in the light body domain until you can gaze at each other joyfully from it, without any distorted fields getting in the way. Only then should you begin working in another domain to restore compatibility.

PART 3
Healing the Family Dynamic

In successful relationships, partners and family members are able to share universal feminine and masculine energy with one another in a balanced way, in all the fields where physical and subtle interactions take place. This includes the normal waking state as well as the sleep state and the death state. Although most people are unaware that these additional states exist, they play an important part in family relationships because they have a significant influence on subtle interactions. The field of sleep has a considerable impact on your ability to sense your physical-material body and experience sensations fully. The field of death influences your ability to experience sexual energy fully and surrender to unconditional joy.

Both of these fields, as well as the normal waking state, exist within everybody in both a dormant and actualized state. The field of sleep and death are dormant while you're awake; the waking state is dormant when you're asleep or dead, and the field of death is dormant while you are in either the normal waking state or the sleep state.

Relationship partners and family members who can share subtle energy and consciousness in all these states will enjoy the benefits of a transcendent relationship, which means they will feel themselves and their family members, empathize with them, and they will be able to share authentic emotions freely. In the next three chapters, we will look at how the normal waking state, the state of sleep, and the state of death influence your family relationships. We will also look at how empathy, emotions, and polarity can be disrupted and how you can restore them—so that you can anticipate the desires and needs of your family members.

You will also learn how you can share prana effortlessly in all states by creating the mutual field of prana. Finally, you will learn to strengthen weak elements and enhance your kidney chi (jing) so that you can share more pleasure, love, and intimacy with the people you love.

— FIVE —

Family Healing

All states, including the waking state, sleep state, and death state, exist within you as fields of subtle energy and consciousness. Interactions on the levels of energy and consciousness take place in these fields even if the people involved are unconscious of them.

In 2016, we began to work with Sebnem, a thirty-two-year-old Turkish woman who lived in Berlin with her husband Howard, an American engineer. They consulted us because Howard had sexual problems, which included a lack of sexual motivation and difficulty maintaining an erection. And Sebnem was unable to express her authentic emotions spontaneously or assert her desires freely—a problem she had been wrestling with since she was a child. Since Sebnem managed a team of social workers, her inability to express herself freely had begun to disrupt her relationship to her teammates. In addition, she had been unable to conceive a child, which depressed her and stressed her relationship with Howard.

We discovered that Howard's problems had their foundation in his death field. And Sebnem's problems were created by a polarity imbalance. We also discovered that Sebnem's polarity problems, which included a disruption of both her back-front polarity and her up-down polarity, were responsible for abdominal cramps and an inability to express her authentic emotions freely, symptoms which she had experienced since puberty.

It's not unusual for a family member whose back-front polarity has become disrupted to have difficulty expressing anger, fear, pain, and joy—the four authentic emotions. In fact, an emotional blockage is one of its most common symptoms.

To compensate for her emotional problem, Sebnem chose to live almost exclusively in her head, which also interfered with her relationship to Howard. In our work, we've learned that this is one way that people deal with the problem; another way is to substitute inauthentic emotions such as arrogance, rage, or contempt for the authentic emotions that they can no longer express freely.

We began by looking into Howard's sexual problems. They had become acute—leading to bouts of self-doubt and irritation that he was having difficulty controlling. By looking into the condition of his subtle field, we discovered that his older brother Jack had projected distorted fields of jealousy at him as well as distorted fields of sexual energy in an unconscious effort to supplant him as his mother's favorite.

It's important to note that the field of death can have a profound influence on a person's sexual energy, their ability to have a satisfying orgasm, and to experience unconditional joy. This is one explanation for why the French refer to orgasm as "the little death."

The brothers had shared the same tiny bedroom until Jack left for the army, which explains why attachments were found mostly in Howard's field of death. By sleeping in such close proximity, the brothers' emotional and mental auras interpenetrated each other at night. As a result of this sleeping arrangement, the negative thoughts and feelings Jack had radiated directly into Howard's subtle field. To overcome the problem, we began by teaching Howard to look inward in order to locate the field of death and then to fill it with prana and bliss. Filling the field of death with prana and bliss restored his confidence, and in a short time, he was able to sustain an erection and satisfy both himself and his wife. Even if you don't suffer from a sexual dysfunction, by locating and clearing out distortions in the field of death, you will enhance your relationships by improving your ability to sense your body, share sexual energy, and experience unconditional joy.

Restoring the field of death had solved Howard's sexual problems. But it didn't solve the long-term problem which was the damage his brother's projections had done to his boundaries. To overcome that problem, it was necessary for Howard to enhance the amount of jing (which is the essence of chi) that radiated through his exceptional meridians. We taught him how to do that a short time later by creating the Boundary Safety Net, which you will find in chapter 17.

EXERCISE: Locating Your Field of Death

To locate the field of death in your subtle field, find a comfortable position with your back straight. Then close your eyes and breathe deeply through your nose for two to three minutes. Continue by asserting, *"It's my intent to go to my personal healing space."* Then bring your awareness to your body, soul, and spirit. Enjoy your healing space for five minutes. Then assert, *"It's my intent to experience the death field within me."* Take five minutes to experience the death field. Then assert, *"It's my intent to center myself in my death field."* Next, assert, *"It's my intent to turn my appropriate senses* (sight, hearing, feeling, etc.) *inward on the level of the death field within me."* It's by turning your appropriate senses inward, on the level of your death field, that you will perceive it in its fullness.

After you've observed the death field and you're satisfied with what you've experienced, count from one to five. When you reach the number five, open your eyes and bring yourself out of the exercise.

EXERCISE: Filling the Field of Death with Prana and Bliss

After you've experienced your field of death, you can fill it with prana and bliss. To begin the exercise, find a comfortable position with your back straight. Then breathe deeply through your nose for two to three minutes. Continue by going to your healing space next. Then bring your awareness to your body, soul, and spirit. Once you're centered, perform the Orgasmic Bliss Mudra (see page 68). Hold the mudra while you assert, *"It's my intent to experience the death field within me."* Take five minutes to experience the death field. Then assert, *"It's my intent to center myself in my death field."* Continue by asserting, *"It's my intent to turn my appropriate organs of perception* (sight, hearing, feeling, etc.) *inward on the level of the death field within me.*" Take five minutes to enjoy the experience. Then assert, *"It's my intent to fill my death field with prana and bliss."* Continue to hold the mudra for five more minutes. Then release it and count from one to five. When you reach the number five, open your eyes and bring yourself out of the meditation.

While Howard performed these exercises, we looked into how he and Sebnem interacted with one another on the subtle levels. Considering their relationship problems, we were surprised to see that they had compatible soul vibrations, core values, and dominant elements. In spite of their natural compatibility and the benefits it gave them, it was clear that Sebnem's polarity problem interfered with Howard's ability to retain an erection as well as her ability to express her emotions freely. In our next session, we began by addressing the problem.

We explained to Sebnem at the beginning of the session that even though energy with universal qualities (prana, chi) plays a special role in family relationships, if it's not in balance, over time polarity problems will develop. These problems can make it difficult, if not impossible, for the afflicted person to share prana with their partner freely.

It's the build-up of energy with individual qualities in a person's subtle field that creates this imbalance. In extreme cases, the build-up of distorted energy can make a family member overly masculine or overly feminine. Since all polarity problems are in fact relationship problems, a polarity problem can affect a person's sexual relationship with their partner as well as their relationship with other family members.

When Balance Has Been Disrupted

When a family member's polarity becomes excessively masculine, which was the case with Sebnem, they can become overly assertive, aggressive, and—in extreme cases—violent. Men and women who've become excessively masculine on the levels of subtle energy leave little room for other people to radiate their energy freely. This can disrupt family relationships because family members will find it difficult to express their emotions or to assert their will and desires freely.

People who are excessively masculine often oppress those dependent on them, particularly women and children. Some feel compelled to control their environment. Others can become arrogant, manipulative, and excessively critical of the people closest to them.

When a family member's polarity becomes excessively feminine, it can make them overly receptive, passive, and—in extreme cases—dependent and/or passive aggressive. People who've become overly feminine can also become hyper-sensitive to the feelings and emotions of others because their surface boundaries have been weakened. Surface boundaries surround all fields within the subtle field, including auric fields, domains, and chakra fields. In order for a person to remain stable on the emotional and mental levels, it's essential that their boundaries remain strong.

There are two forms of polarity that have a significant influence on the health of intimate relationships: back-front polarity and up-down polarity. We will look at back-front polarity first.

Back-Front Polarity

Back-front polarity is extremely important because it regulates your ability to express anger, fear, pain, and joy—your four authentic emotions. It also affects your self-confidence, self-esteem, and your ability to create and maintain a strong personal identity.

Let's take a moment to look at how back-front polarity can influence your ability to express authentic emotions. According to the principles of polarity, the back of your body is masculine in relationship to the front, which is feminine. Back-front polarity is the same for men, women, and children.

The reason for this is simple to understand. In a person's non-physical field, the movement of masculine energy is strongest through the main masculine meridian, the governor, in the back of the body. The movement of feminine energy is strongest through the main feminine meridian, the conceptual, in the front of the body (see figure 10: Back-Front Polarity, page 84).

To fully understand how back-front polarity influences your emotional life, you first need to know that there are two types of emotions: authentic emotions and inauthentic emotions. Emotions that are authentic have their foundation in prana moving upward through the governor meridian, in the back of your body.

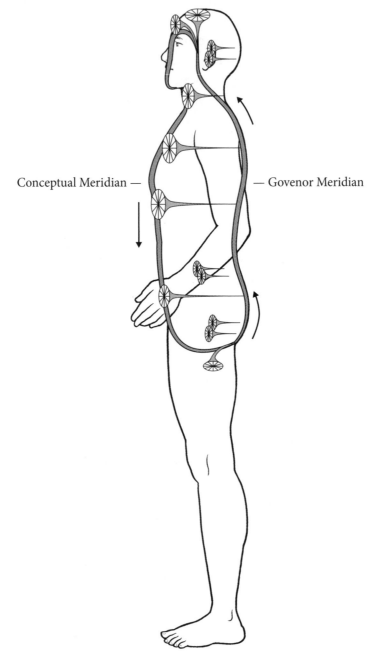

Conceptual Meridian —   — Govenor Meridian

Figure 10: Back-Front Polarity

Emotions that are inauthentic have their foundation in fields of energy with individual qualities that have become trapped in your non-physical field. When prana (chi) emerging from the base of your spine flows upward through the governor meridian without disruption, no authentic emotions will emerge. It's only when attachments to fields of energy with individual qualities and external projections have blocked the flow of energy through the governor meridian that an authentic emotion will be produced.

If you turn your attention to figure 10: Back-Front Polarity, page 84, you can see that the main masculine meridian, the governor, passes through the back of the seven traditional chakra gates. When prana flowing through the governor meridian is prevented from moving upward in the vicinity of a chakra gate, it will be forced to move forward. When that energy reaches the middle of the chakra gate, a point which corresponds to the mid-point of your physical-material body, its polarity, which was masculine (because it was in the back of the body), will be reversed, and it will become feminine. That's the exact moment when an authentic emotion will emerge.

Anger emerges when prana is forced through the second chakra gate; fear emerges when prana is forced through the third chakra gate; pain emerges when prana is forced through the fourth chakra gate, and joy emerges when prana is forced through the fifth chakra gate.

Human beings have evolved the ability to express the four authentic emotions as soon as they emerge by crying, yelling, screaming, etc., as well as through their eyes and facial musculature. Expressing an authentic emotion spontaneously will create a feeling of satisfaction which indicates that the pent-up emotional energy has reached the organs of expression in the head and a healthy flow of prana through the governor meridian has been restored.

If the emotional energy isn't expressed spontaneously, it will continue to flow forward, through the front of your chakra gate into the auric field, where it will get trapped. No amount of crying, screaming, or shouting after the fact will transmute this residual emotional energy and release it. Emotional energy which has not been expressed spontaneously will become part of the dense, qualified energy known as karmic baggage, which is deposited in the auric fields surrounding personal body space.[9]

Sebnem was unable to express authentic emotions because her father had wanted a son. And rather than accepting her, he projected distorted fields of energy into her field. These projections blocked her femininity by blocking the functions of her second through fifth chakras. To restore her back-front polarity, we taught Sebnem to perform the following series of exercises. We also taught them to Howard since her condition had impacted his ability to express himself freely and to perform sexually.

Each exercise will enhance your ability to express one of the four authentic emotions—anger, fear, pain, and joy—freely. Sebnem practiced them regularly and they restored her back-front polarity. If you have difficulty expressing any of the four authentic emotions, perform the appropriate exercise, and it will do the same for you.

Before you begin to perform the exercises, it's important to recognize two things. The first is that by restoring a healthy flow of energy, authentic emotions serve as safety valves. These safety valves evolved along with your organs of expression to bring back-front polarity into a healthy balance and restore relationship when it's been disrupted by blockages and external projections.

The second is that emotions are a function of polarity, not gender. This means that emotions are feminine—that's all! It doesn't mean that women are inherently more emotional than men. Women may be subject to different hormonal and cultural influences than men, but there's nothing in their energy fields that makes them inherently more emotional. All we can say with confidence is that when prana has been forced forward and enters the front half of your subtle field, an authentic emotion will emerge.[10]

EXERCISE: The Authentic Anger Meditation

Anger is a normal reaction to the disruption of intimate relationships. In the Authentic Anger Meditation, you will enhance your ability to express anger when it's appropriate by activating your second chakra, centering yourself in your second chakra field, and then filling your second chakra field with prana. After that, you will continue to fill your right and left kwas with prana. An inability to express anger was

Sebnem's most pressing problem, one that was quickly resolved once she began to practice the Authentic Anger Meditation.

To begin the exercise, find a comfortable position with your back straight. Close your eyes and breathe deeply through your nose for two to three minutes. Then go to your healing space and bring your awareness to your body, soul, and spirit. Enjoy the process for five minutes. Then assert, *"It's my intent to activate my second chakra."* Continue by asserting, *"It's my intent to center myself in my second chakra field."* Once you're centered, assert, *"It's my intent to fill my second chakra field with prana."* Take two to three minutes to enjoy the process.

Then assert, *"It's my intent to fill my right and left kwas with prana"* (see figure 2: Taoist Subtle Anatomy, page 14). Take ten minutes more to fill your second chakra field and kwas with prana. Then count from one to five. When you reach the number five, open your eyes and bring yourself out of the meditation. Repeat as needed.

To enhance your ability to express authentic fear, you can use the same exercise. Simply substitute your third chakra and chakra field for your second chakra and chakra field and your two midriff cavities for your two kwas while you are centered in your personal healing space.

To enhance your ability to express authentic pain, you can use the same exercise. Simply substitute your fourth chakra and chakra field for your third chakra and chakra field and your two armpit cavities for your two midriff cavities while you are centered in your personal healing space.

To enhance your ability to express authentic joy, you can use the same exercise. Simply substitute your fifth chakra and chakra field for your fourth chakra and chakra field and your Eye of Brahma for your two armpit cavities while you are centered in your personal healing space.

— SIX —
Caring for One Another

There is another form of polarity that we call up-down polarity. It plays an important part in partnership and family relationships because it enhances a family member's ability to share universal energy and its essence—and it supports sexual intimacy and physical coitus.

Most of Sebnem's emotional issues were resolved by restoring her back-front polarity. But it was a disruption in Sebnem's up-down polarity that contributed to her cramps and her difficulty conceiving a child.

Another couple, Alan and Serena, who had been together for six years, consulted us in 2016. Both had been divorced. Their fifteen-year-old son, Dennis, had a non-binary gender expression and had been creating what his stepfather labeled "outlandish outfits" to wear to school. Within minutes of their arrival, Alan began to complain that his stepson was out of control and needed to be disciplined. He believed that Dennis had been influenced by websites and social media—and that he was moving in the wrong direction by acting and dressing the way he did.

Although there was nothing fundamentally wrong with his choices, we quickly recognized that Dennis felt abandoned by his natural father and was rebelling against the energetic environment that his stepfather had created.

The crux of Dennis's problem, on the subtle level, was an imbalance in his up-down polarity. It had been disrupted by his biological parents who had divorced when he was six. A long and divisive court battle ensued for custody of Dennis and his brother Kevin. The court gave primary custody to his mother, Serena. But by then the family dynamic had been poisoned and so had Dennis's relationship to his natural father, who felt so diminished that he moved one thousand miles away and rarely saw his two boys after that.

We began by teaching Dennis to restore his up-down polarity.

Up-Down Polarity

In male-female relationships, men are masculine by the second chakra and feminine by the heart chakra. Women are feminine by the second chakra and masculine by the heart chakra. This principle applies to same-sex couples and transgender partnerships. That's because in all long-term, intimate relationships, one partner will be more assertive by their heart chakra and more receptive by their second chakra, and the other partner will be more assertive by their second chakra and more receptive by their heart chakra when they interact with one another.

Figure 11 shows how up-down polarity plays out in a long-term, intimate relationship (see figure 11: Up-Down Polarity, page 91). The arrows indicate the movement of subtle energy between two partners. When the assertive partner has been stimulated by their more receptive partner, the assertive partner will react, as a function of up-down polarity, by asserting energy forward from their second chakra. If their partner is receptive, they will respond, as a function of up-down polarity, by drawing energy from their auric field inward, through their second chakra. The enhanced flow of subtle energy inward will activate the receptive partner's second chakra and enhance its function. Once the chakra has become active, more energy will flow downward through the conceptual meridian, in the front of the receptive partner's body towards their first chakra, at the base of their spine.

When the enhanced flow of energy reaches the center of their first chakra, its polarity will be reversed, and it will become masculine because it has entered the back of personal body space, which is masculine in relationship to the front, which is feminine. At the same time, the receptive partner's first chakra will become active, and they will feel more secure and comfortable in their body.

Subtle energy, which activated the receptive partner's first chakra, will continue to move up the back of their energy field. The increased flow of energy will empower them because personal power is largely determined by how much energy can flow upward through the governor meridian.

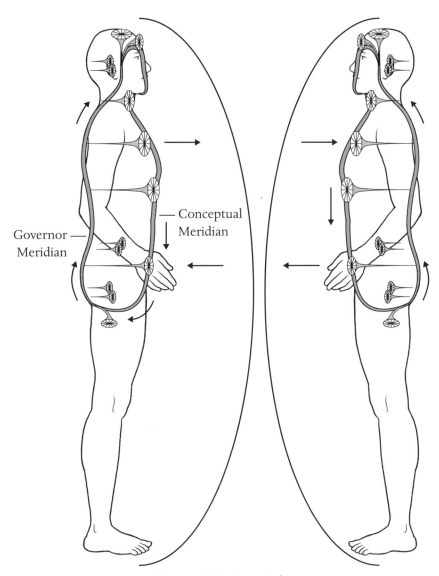

Figure 11: Up-Down Polarity

Once the energy reaches their heart chakra (which in a receptive partner is polarized masculine), the chakra will become active. That will enhance the flow of energy through it, which will create a sympathetic reaction that will stimulate their partner's heart chakra and make them more receptive.

Once their partner's heart chakra has become active, more energy will radiate down the conceptual meridian in the front of their body. If there are no blockages which disrupt the movement of energy, it will reach the front of the second chakra and activate it. That will complete the circuit of energy in an intimate relationship, created by up-down polarity.

In a relationship where up-down polarity is in balance, the receptive partner will be empowered and become more self-confident. However, because of up-down polarity, a receptive partner will also seek to be embraced by the relationship. If they're not embraced, the receptive partner will often feel disappointed.

The assertive partner will also be deeply affected by up-down polarity. When it's in balance, the assertive partner will be more empathetic and gentle and more receptive to universal feminine energy. However, even if they're committed to their partner, individuals who take on the primary assertive role usually have a deep need to retain their individuality because the back of their energy field remains outside the polar relationship created by up-down polarity.

Even so—it should be clear that when up-down polarity is in balance, energetic interactions between family members will enhance pleasure, love, intimacy, and joy, which all are necessary ingredients for a successful relationship.

To heal Sebnem's polarity problem, we taught her to perform the Nine Cavity Meditation. We taught the same meditation to Dennis and his parents. We did this in order to restore Dennis's polarity and to restore the relationship his family members in the household had to one another.

The importance of the Nine Cavity Meditation lies in its ability to restore a healthy flow of chi (prana) through the subtle field and to balance the flow between the thirteen chakras in body space as well as the nine cavities that compose the microcosmic circuit.

EXERCISE: The Nine Cavity Meditation

The nine cavities you will be working with in the Nine Cavity Meditation include the lower, middle, and upper dantians as well as the two kwas, two midriff cavities, and two armpit cavities (see figure 2: Taoist Subtle Anatomy, page 14).

To begin the meditation, find a comfortable position with your back straight. Then close your eyes and breathe deeply through your nose for two to three minutes. Once you're relaxed, assert, *"It's my intent to go to my personal healing space."* Once you've experienced your personal healing space, bring your awareness to your body, soul, and spirit. Enjoy the process for five minutes. Then bring the tip of your tongue to the top of your mouth directly behind your teeth. In Taoism, this is known as closing the gate. Once your tongue is in position, mentally assert, *"It's my intent to center myself in my lower dantian."* Take a moment to experience the shift. Then mentally assert in words not thoughts, *"It's my intent to fill my lower dantian with chi."* Enjoy the process for two to three minutes. Then continue in the same way with the middle and upper dantian. After you've filled your middle and upper dantians with chi, assert, *"It's my intent to center myself in my right and left kwas."* Then assert, *"It's my intent to fill my right and left kwas with chi."* Enjoy the process for an additional two to three minutes. Then use the same method to center yourself and fill your right and left midriff cavities with chi. After a short pause, center yourself in your right and left armpit cavities and continue by filling them with chi.

Once you've filled your two armpit cavities with chi, relax and enjoy the shift you experience for another ten minutes. Then count from one to five. When you reach the number five, open your eyes and bring yourself out of the meditation. By practicing the exercise every day for a month, you will bring your up-down polarity into a noticeably healthier balance.

The Problem of Reversed Polarity

Reversed polarity is caused by an extreme disruption of up-down polarity. Reversed polarity in a family member who has taken on the primary assertive role will cause the afflicted person to become feminine by their second chakra and masculine by their heart chakra. Reversed polarity in a family member who has taken on the primary receptive role will cause the afflicted person to become masculine by their second chakra and feminine by their heart chakra.

Randy's self-limiting core values and the divisive environment it had created in his family had created polarity problems for his two children. As you learned earlier, his son William had suffered most from the family dynamic. His father's projections had disrupted the functions of his second and fourth chakras. This in turn had disrupted his polarity to such an extent that it had become reversed.

Experience has taught us that, to heal the condition, it's essential to heal the subtle organs that have the greatest influence on the balance of up-down polarity. These include the three kandas located in the back of body space and the second and fourth chakras. The first kanda is located behind the first chakra at the base of the spine. The second kanda is located behind the heart chakra between the shoulder blades, and the third kanda is located behind the back of the crown chakra in the rear of the head (see figure 12: The Three Kandas, page 95).

The kandas are important because they serve as energetic hubs that distribute prana from resource fields to the organs of the subtle field—particularly the seven traditional chakras and the major meridians that connect them. In the next two exercises you will restore the kandas and the second and fourth chakra fields to radiant good health. In that way, you will restore your up-down polarity to a healthy balance if it's been reversed.

The first exercise you will perform is called the Enhanced Kanda Technique. The second is called the Second and Fourth Chakra Meditation. We taught these exercises to William as soon as we met him. Changes began almost immediately. And within six weeks, he brought their up-down polarity into a healthy balance.

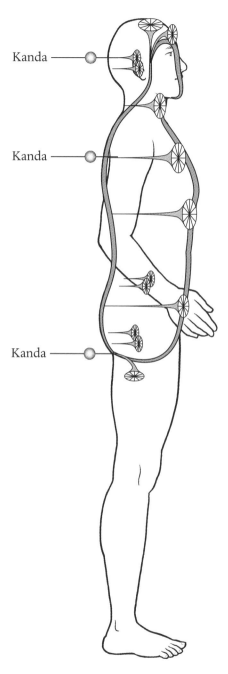

Figure 12: The Three Kandas

EXERCISE: The Enhanced Kanda Technique

In this exercise, you will fill your three kandas with prana. This will not only enhance the functions of the kandas; it will restore the flow of prana up the governor meridian and down the conceptual meridian.

To begin the meditation, find a comfortable position with your back straight. Then close your eyes and breathe deeply through your nose for two to three minutes. Once you're relaxed, assert, *"It's my intent to go to my personal healing space."* Once you've experienced your personal healing space, bring your awareness to your body, soul, and spirit. Enjoy the process for five minutes. Then assert, *"It's my intent to center myself in my first kanda at the base of my spine"* (see figure 12: The Three Kandas, page 95). Once you're centered, assert, *"It's my intent to fill my first kanda with prana."* Take five minutes to enjoy the process. Then assert, *"It's my intent to center myself in my second kanda behind my heart chakra."* Once you're centered, assert, *"It's my intent to fill my second kanda with prana."* Take five minutes to fill the kanda with prana. Then assert, *"It's my intent to center myself in my third kanda in back of my crown chakra in the rear of the head."* Then assert, *"It's my intent to fill my third kanda with prana."* Take ten minutes more to enjoy the process. Then count from one to five. When you reach the number five, open your eyes and bring yourself out of the exercise. Once you've performed the Enhanced Kanda Technique, we suggest you perform the Second and Fourth Chakra Meditation.

EXERCISE: The Second and Fourth Chakra Meditation

To begin the exercise, sit in a comfortable position with your back straight. Then close your eyes and breathe deeply through your nose for two to three minutes. Once you're relaxed, assert, *"It's my intent to go to my personal healing space."* Once you've experienced your personal healing space, bring your awareness to your body, soul, and spirit. Enjoy the process for five minutes. Then assert, *"It's my intent to activate my second chakra."* Continue by asserting, *"It's my intent to center myself in my second chakra field."* Once you're centered in your second chakra field, assert, *"It's my intent to activate my fourth chakra."* Continue by asserting, *"It's my intent to center myself in my fourth chakra field."* Once you're centered in your fourth chakra field, assert, *"It's my intent to fill my second and fourth chakra fields with prana."* Take ten more minutes to enjoy the process. Then count from one to five. When you reach the number five, open your eyes and bring yourself out of the meditation.

Practice the Second and Fourth Chakra Meditation along with the Enhanced Kanda Technique regularly—and, in a short time, you will overcome the issue of reversed polarity.

The Three Fields of Empathy

Empathy is the ability to share the feelings, needs, and desires of other people. It's one of the key ingredients of successful relationships because it helps family members understand the perspectives, needs, and intentions of their loved ones.

On the subtle levels, every person has three fields of empathy. They're resource fields through which energy can be exchanged selflessly without the "I" or the ego getting in the way. The three fields of empathy are known as the Public Field of Empathy, the Personal Field of Empathy, and the Universal Field of Empathy.

To experience more empathy for your family members, you must begin by enhancing your empathy for Universal Consciousness, the source of empathy and the universal qualities that make relationships so joyful and satisfying. The next step is to increase your empathy for yourself. Only after that can you enhance your empathy for other people.

In the following pages, you will use a technique we designed specially to enhance your empathy for Universal Consciousness. After that, you can use the same technique to enhance your empathy for yourself and your loved ones.

We taught this exercise to many of the family members we worked with. Andrew used it to restore his empathy and to enhance his ability to feel himself and his family members. And Randy used it to enhance his empathy and understanding for his wife and children.

EXERCISE: The Enhanced Empathy Technique

To enhance your empathy for Universal Consciousness, find a comfortable position with your back straight. Close your eyes and breathe deeply through your nose for two to three minutes. Then count backward from five to one and from ten to one. Continue by asserting, *"It's my intent to go to my personal healing space."* Once you've experienced your personal healing space, bring your awareness to your body, soul, and spirit. Enjoy the process for five minutes. Then assert, *"It's my intent to center myself in my universal field of empathy."* Continue by asserting, *"It's my intent to turn my appropriate organs of perception inward on the level of the universal field of empathy."* Take a moment to enjoy the shift. Then assert, *"It's my intent to fill my universal field of empathy with prana."* Take fifteen minutes to fill your universal field with prana. Then count from one to five. When you reach the number five, open your eyes and bring yourself out of the meditation. Continue to practice the exercise every day for two weeks. Then repeat as needed.

EXERCISE: Enhancing Empathy for Yourself

In this exercise, you will center yourself in the personal field of empathy and fill it with prana. By doing that, you will enhance your empathy for yourself. That will enhance your self-awareness, self-esteem, and ability to experience pleasure without judgment.

To begin, find a comfortable position with your back straight. Close your eyes and breathe deeply through your nose for two to three minutes. Then count backward from five to one and from ten to one. Once you're relaxed, assert, *"It's my intent to go to my personal healing space."* Once you've experienced your personal healing space, bring your awareness to your body, soul, and spirit. Enjoy the process for five minutes. Then assert, *"It's my intent to center myself in my personal field of empathy."* Continue by asserting, *"It's my intent to turn my appropriate organs of perception inward on the level of my personal field of empathy."* Take a few moments to enjoy the shift. Then assert, *"It's my intent to fill my personal field of empathy with prana."* Continue to fill your personal field of empathy with prana for fifteen minutes more. Then count from one to five. When you reach the number five, open your eyes and bring yourself out of the meditation. Continue to perform the exercise every day for two weeks. Then repeat as needed.

EXERCISE: Enhancing Empathy for Your Partner and Children

By centering yourself in the public field of empathy and filling it with prana, you will enhance your empathy for your partner and children. That in turn will enhance your respect for your family members and for universal feminine energy.

To begin, find a comfortable position with your back straight. Close your eyes and breathe deeply through your nose for two to three minutes. Then count backward from five to one and from ten to one. Once you're relaxed, assert, *"It's my intent to go to my personal healing space."* Once you've experienced your personal healing space, bring your awareness to your body, soul, and spirit. Enjoy the process for five minutes. Then assert, *"It's my intent to center myself in my public field of empathy."* Continue by asserting, *"It's my intent to turn my appropriate organs of perception inward on the level of my public field of empathy."* Take a few moments to enjoy the shift. Then assert, *"It's my intent to fill my public field of empathy with prana."* Take fifteen minutes more to fill your public field of empathy with prana. Then count from one to five. When you reach the number five, open your eyes and bring yourself out of the meditation. Continue to practice the exercise every day for two weeks. Then repeat as needed.

— SEVEN —
Strengthening Your Relationship

In this chapter, we will address the issues that make living together more joyful and satisfying. To that end, we will delve into the mysteries of the microcosmic circuit, one of the most important energetic systems in your subtle field. After that, we will provide you and your family members with exercises that will enhance the flow of prana (chi) and jing (the essence of chi) through your microcosmic circuit. That in turn will enable you and your family members to share prana and jing effortlessly—so that you can experience greater pleasure, intimacy and joy with one another.

The Microcosmic Circuit

Both Taoists and Yogic adepts recognize the importance of the microcosmic circuit. They tell us that it plays an essential part in two important activities. It regulates the flow of chi (prana) and jing through your subtle energy field. And it maintains a healthy balance of polarity in both your subtle energy field and physical-material body. Both influence your ability to share your feelings and emotions with your family members. In addition, when functioning healthfully, the microcosmic circuit protects your subtle field from intrusions of distorted energy.

We've learned that it's most effective to include the three dantians and their neighboring cavities, the governor and conceptual meridians, as well as all the chakras in body space when working with the microcosmic circuit because each of these organs has an important function related to family relationships and personal well-being (see figure 13: The Microcosmic Circuit, page 103).

The microcosmic circuit can regulate the flow of chi (prana) and jing through the subtle energy field because the perineum, where the first chakra is located, has a negative polarity, while the crown of the head, where the seventh chakra is located, has a positive polarity. By circulating chi and jing between these two poles, the microcosmic circuit increases their strength because the differential draws additional chi and jing from resource fields through the kandas into the microcosmic circuit. From the microcosmic circuit, both chi and jing are then circulated through the remaining organs of your subtle energy field, including the exceptional meridians (to learn more about them go to chapter 8), auric fields, and minor energy centers. Although there is great flexibility to the way the microcosmic circuit transmits chi and jing when it's functioning healthfully, it's the water cycle that will enhance family relationships the most.

The Water Cycle

Taoist texts tell us that the water cycle circulates chi and jing up the back of your body, through the governor meridian, and down the front of your body through the conceptual meridian. We've discovered that the movement of chi and jing in this way has a profound effect on family relationships for several reasons. It enhances intuition and relaxes the nerves along the spine which can have a significant effect on your ability to make life-affirming decisions. It integrates the functions of the three dantians and their subsidiary cavities including the kwas, midriff cavities, and armpit cavities. And it distributes chi and jing most readily to the chakras in body space as well as those above and below it.

In the body of this chapter, you will learn to enhance the functions of your microcosmic circuit. But before we can do that, it's important for you to know more about its structure and function, especially the structure and function of the meridians that transmit chi and jing and serve as its boundaries.

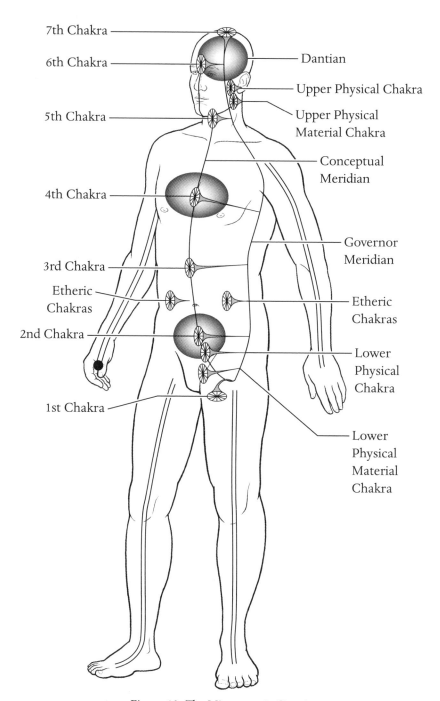

Figure 13: The Microcosmic Circuit

Meridians

Structurally, meridians are streams of energy that connect the chakras, dantians, and minor energy centers to one another. Although functionally the meridians correspond to the veins and arteries of the circulatory system, which distribute blood and life-nurturing nutrients throughout the physical-material body, structurally they more closely resemble currents of water and/or air found in the earth's oceans and atmosphere. Their flexible structure makes it possible for them to maintain the flow of energy with universal qualities and its essence, jing, within the microcosmic circuit at healthy levels. This in turn will keep back-front and up-down polarity in balance. You will learn more about jing and how it influences your well-being and family relationships in the next chapter.

Individually and collectively, meridians have two additional functions that bear directly on the health of your family relationships. They connect the organs of the human energy system together, which integrates the functions of your body, soul, and spirit. And they distribute energy to the auric fields and from there into the physical-material body, which will keep them filled with life-affirming energy and jing.

Although there are at least ten major meridians and eight exceptional meridians that transmit jing, as well as thousands of minor meridians in the subtle energy field, the governor and conceptual meridians have the most influence on family relationships. These two meridians connect the organs of the microcosmic circuit together, and they serve as its external boundaries.

Governor and Conceptual Meridians

The governor meridian is the most important masculine meridian in the human energy system. It originates at the perineum, at the base of the spine, and extends upward along the spine to the seventh chakra located at the crown of your head. The masculine poles of the seven traditional chakra gates are connected to it as well as the three dantians. In addition, the governor meridian has a functional connection to the remaining chakras in body space and the cavities that are located alongside the dantians.

The conceptual meridian is the most important feminine meridian in the human energy system. It originates at your brow and makes its way down the front surface of personal body space to a point just behind your sexual organs. The female poles of the seven traditional chakras are connected to it as well as the three dantians. The conceptual meridian has a functional connection to the remaining chakras in body space and the cavities that are located alongside the dantians.

In the following series of exercises, you will stimulate the microcosmic circuit in order to increase the amount of prana and jing flowing through it. By doing that, you will enhance the quantity of energy you can share with your family members. For best results, we've found that it's best to do this in steps. The first step will be to enhance the flow of prana (chi) and jing through the main masculine meridian, the governor, and the male poles of the chakras connected to it. You can do this by performing the Governor Meridian Meditation.

In the Governor Meridian Meditation, you will enhance the flow of prana and jing up your back by activating the back of the seven traditional chakra gates. That will enhance your personal power as well as your stability, mental clarity, self-confidence, and your ability to feel and express your authentic feelings and emotions.

EXERCISE: The Governor Meridian Meditation

To begin the Governor Meridian Meditation, find a comfortable position with your back straight. Then close your eyes and breathe deeply through your nose for two to three minutes. Count backward from ten to one and from five to one. Then assert, *"It's my intent to go to my personal healing space."* Once you've experienced your personal healing space, bring your awareness to your body, soul, and spirit. Enjoy the process for five minutes. Then assert, *"It's my intent to bring my mental attention to the back of my first chakra gate at the base of my spine."* Once you've brought your mental attention to the back of your first chakra gate, breathe into it. That will activate the chakra further by bringing prana, which is entering your subtle energy field on each inhalation, to the back of the chakra gate. Continue to breathe into the back of the first chakra gate for two to three minutes while you enjoy the chakra's enhanced vibration. Then breathe normally again and move your mental attention slowly upward until it reaches the back of your second chakra gate. Once it's reached the back of the chakra gate, assert, *"It's my intent to bring my mental attention to the back of my second chakra gate."* Breathe into the back of the second chakra for two to three minutes while you enjoy the effects. Continue in the same way with the back of your third, fourth, fifth, sixth, and seventh chakras.

Once you've activated the back of the seven traditional chakra gates, assert, *"It's my intent to center myself in my chakra fields on the level of my seven traditional chakras."* Take fifteen minutes to enjoy the experience. After fifteen minutes, count from one to five. When you reach the number five, open your eyes and bring yourself out of the meditation. Repeat the exercise regularly until you can freely share universal masculine energy with your partner and family members.

After Sebnem brought her up-down polarity into balance, we taught her how to perform the Governor Meridian Meditation. It had an immediate effect. It strengthened the universal masculine qualities that had been suppressed by her father's projections—and it helped her to maintain a healthy balance of masculine and feminine energy in her subtle energy field. After practicing the meditation regularly for a month, she began to assert her feelings and emotions more freely and to take a more assertive role in the bedroom.

We taught the same meditation to Dennis in order to help him achieve a more balanced polarity. We didn't want him to change his gender orientation. For that reason, we taught him to perform the Conceptual Meridian Meditation as well. By performing both exercises, he restored the balance of his up-down polarity to its natural state. In a short time, he felt more confident to express his natural gender identity and resist the judgment of other people.

EXERCISE: The Conceptual Meridian Meditation

In this meditation, you will enhance the flow of feminine energy through your conceptual meridian by activating the female poles of the chakra gates connected to it. By doing that, you will do several things that will enhance the health of your relationships. You will increase the amount of receptive (feminine) energy you have available by enhancing the flow of prana down the front of your body. And you will enhance your ability to share the life-affirming qualities associated with universal feminine energy.

To begin the meditation, find a comfortable position with your back straight. Then close your eyes and breathe deeply through your nose for two to three minutes. Count backward from ten to one and from five to one. Then assert, *"It's my intent to go to my personal healing space."* Once you've experienced your personal healing space, bring your awareness to your body, soul, and spirit. Enjoy the process for five minutes. Then assert, *"It's my intent to bring my mental attention to the front of my seventh chakra gate at the crown of my head."* Once your mental attention is focused on the gate, breathe into it. That will activate the chakra further by bringing prana entering your subtle energy field on each inhalation to the gate. Continue to breathe into the front of the seventh chakra gate for one to two minutes while you enjoy the chakra's enhanced vibration. Then breathe normally again and move your mental attention downward along the meridian until it reaches the front of your sixth chakra gate by your brow. As soon as it has reached the chakra gate, assert, *"It's my intent to bring my mental attention to the front of my sixth chakra gate."* Breathe into the front of the sixth chakra gate for two to three minutes. Then continue in the same way with the front of your fifth, fourth, third, second, and first chakras.

Once you've activated the front of the seven traditional chakras, assert, *"It's my intent to center myself in my chakra fields on the level of my seven traditional chakras."* Take fifteen minutes to enjoy the experience. After fifteen minutes, count from one to five. When you reach the number five, open your eyes and bring yourself out of the meditation.

We recommend that you practice the meditation regularly until you can share universal feminine energy with your partner freely.

EXERCISE: The Microcosmic Circuit Meditation

We've taught the Microcosmic Circuit Meditation to many of the family members we worked with because it enhances a man's receptivity and makes him more gentle and affectionate. And it empowers women and enhances their awareness of their inherent personal rights.

We made a special point of teaching this exercise to Wendy and Charlie so that they could create a healthy bond with Tim and provide him with the space he needed, on the subtle levels, to create a healthy identity.

Wendy and Charlie continued to perform the exercise for several weeks. And although we didn't meet with them again, we did receive a Christmas card from them. In the card, they explained that they were all well and that their relationship with Tim had become one of their greatest joys.

In the Microcosmic Circuit Meditation, you will combine what you've learned in the previous two meditations. You will also "Close the Gate" by bringing the tip of your tongue behind your upper teeth. Closing the gate will enhance the flow of prana between your conceptual and governor meridians. That in turn will help ground you—which will make it easier for you to stay centered in your authentic mind for extended periods of time.

To begin the meditation, find a comfortable position with your back straight. Close your eyes and breathe deeply through your nose for two to three minutes. Then assert, *"It's my intent to go to my personal healing space."* Once you've experienced your personal healing space, bring your awareness to your body, soul, and spirit. Enjoy the process for five minutes. Then close the gate by bringing the tip of your tongue to the top of your mouth directly behind your teeth. Hold your tongue in that position and in words mentally assert, *"It's my intent to bring my mental attention to the back of my first chakra gate at the base of my spine."* Continue by breathing into the back of the first chakra gate for one to two minutes. Then breathe normally again and move your mental attention slowly upward until it reaches the back of your second chakra gate. Continue by asserting, *"It's my intent to bring my mental attention to the back of my second chakra gate."* Then breathe into the back of the second chakra for one to two minutes. Continue in the same way with the back of your third, fourth, fifth, sixth, and seventh chakras.

After you've activated the masculine pole of your seven chakra gates, assert, *"It's my intent to bring my mental attention to the front of my seventh chakra gate at the crown of my head."* Continue by breathing into the chakra gate for one to two minutes. Then breathe normally again and move your mental attention slowly downward until you reach your brow where the feminine pole of the sixth chakra gate is located. Breathe into it for one to two minutes. Then continue in the same way until you've activated the feminine pole of all the seven traditional chakras.

Once you've activated the front of the seven traditional chakra gates, assert, *"It's my intent to center myself in my chakra fields on the level of my seven traditional chakras."* Take fifteen minutes more to enjoy the experience. After fifteen minutes, count from one to five. When you reach the number five, open your eyes and bring yourself out of the meditation. Repeat as needed.

After releasing negative core values and replacing them with core values that were life-affirming, we taught Simon and Irene to perform the Microcosmic Circuit Meditation. By performing the meditation for just over a month, Simon and Irene were able to share their feelings and the responsibilities of parenting more easily. Their success motivated them to continue—and, within another two months of practice, Simon no longer felt more entitled than other people, especially women, and Irene no longer resented the men in her life.

They were so enthusiastic with the changes they'd experienced that they chose to take the next step in the process by learning to release blockages in their kandas. These were blockages that had the potential to block the flow of prana entering their microcosmic circuit from their chakra fields.

Kandas and Prana

There are three kandas that influence the health of the microcosmic circuit. They are hubs that distribute energy from the chakra fields to the conceptual and governor meridians and from there throughout the subtle energy field. They are closely related to both the dantians and their six complementary cavities. The lower kanda is located directly behind the first chakra and is associated with the lower dantian. The middle kanda is located directly behind the fourth chakra and is associated with the middle dantian, and the upper kanda is located directly behind the seventh chakra and is associated with the upper dantian (see figure 12: The Three Kandas, page 95).

To release blockages in the kandas and restore the flow of energy from your chakra fields, you will perform two exercises. In the first exercise you will gaze at your partner from each of your dantians, beginning with the lower dantian. By gazing from each of the dantians, you will be able to determine if you have a blockage in the kanda connected to it.

If there are blockages in any of your kandas, then you won't connect in a satisfying way or experience a deeper sense of well-being when you gaze at your partner from the dantians. Instead, you will become anxious, frustrated, and/or irritated. If there are no blockages in the kanda, your breathing will get deeper and your muscles will relax. In addition, thoughts will give way to a deep sense of well-being that will bring you closer to one other.

If you find a blockage, you can use the Prana Box Technique to release distorted fields of energy that have blocked the functions of the kanda. By releasing the blockage in the kanda, prana will flow more freely into the dantian and the microcosmic circuit—and you will be able to share that energy with your partner.

The prana box is similar to the bliss box that you used to release blockages in your domains. The only difference is that instead of using bliss to create the box and to release the blockages, you will use prana.

Before we begin, it's important to note that even though energy with individual qualities has the power to create blockages and cause disease, it's far weaker than prana. This means that prana can release energy with individual qualities when used effectively, no matter how dense and distorted the energy with individual qualities has become.

We taught the Dantian Eye Scan and the prana box to Sebnem and Howard, as well as to most of the families that suffered from projections of distorted energy. We did that because these two exercises, when used in tandem, provide a simple and effective way for people new to deep family healing to release blockages in the kandas and restore the functions of the microcosmic circuit.

EXERCISE: The Dantian Eye Scan

In this exercise, you will gaze at your partner from the lower dantian to determine if there are blockages in the kanda associated with it. Once you've performed the exercise from the lower dantian, you can use the same technique to determine if there are blockages in the kandas associated with the middle and upper dantians.

The first time they performed the exercise, Simon and Irene had difficulty gazing at one another from the lower dantian and, according to Irene, the longer she gazed at her husband, the more detached from her body and her feelings she became. Her reaction led us to the conclusion that the couple had developed a dominant-submissive pattern that was activated whenever they had a major disagreement. It also motivated us to look deeper into the condition of Irene's subtle field. On closer inspection, we discovered that she had suffered a significant trauma in childhood and, when we brought this to her attention, she confessed that she had been sexually abused by her high school swimming coach. In chapter 12, you will learn how Irene overcame the trauma and how you can do the same.

To begin the Dantian Eye Scan, sit facing your partner close enough to hold hands. Keep your backs straight. Then breathe deeply through the nose for two to three minutes. Once you're relaxed, assert, *"It's my intent to go to my personal healing space."* Once you've experienced your personal healing space, bring your awareness to your body, soul, and spirit. Enjoy the process for five minutes. Then assert, *"It's my intent to center myself in my lower dantian."* Take a few moments to enjoy the shift. Then assert, *"It's my intent to turn my appropriate organs of perception inward on the level of my lower dantian."*

When you're ready to continue, open your eyes and gaze at your partner. Continue to gaze at one another for five minutes. Then count from one to five. When you reach the number five, open your eyes and bring yourself out of the exercise.

EXERCISE: Releasing Blockages in the Kandas

If you've found blockages in any of the kandas, you can use the prana box to release them. In the following exercise, you will use the prana box to release blockages in your lower kanda. Once you feel confident, you can use the same exercise to release blockages located in both the middle and upper kandas.

To begin the exercise, find a comfortable position with your back straight. Breathe deeply through your nose for two to three minutes. Then assert, *"It's my intent to go to my personal healing space."* Once you've experienced your personal healing space, bring your awareness to your body, soul, and spirit. Enjoy the process for five minutes. Then assert, *"It's my intent to center myself in my lower kanda."* Continue by asserting, *"It's my intent to turn my appropriate organs of perception inward on the level of my lower kanda."* Once you've turned your organs of perception inward, assert, *"It's my intent to surround the most distorted field of energy in my lower kanda with a prana box."* As soon as you can sense and/or see the box, assert, *"It's my intent to fill the box with prana and release all the distorted fields of energy within it."* Don't do anything after that. Prana will fill the box you've created and release the distorted field automatically.

Some of you may experience a sense of relief and/or a pop when prana fills the box. Both indicate that the distorted field within the prana box has been released and prana has filled the empty space.

Once the distorted field has been released, release the prana box. Then count from one to five. When you reach the number five, open your eyes and bring yourself out of the exercise.

There's often more than one blockage that disrupts the flow of prana from a kanda into the microcosmic circuit. Therefore, you may have to repeat the exercise several times. Each time you repeat the exercise, release the most distorted field of energy. In this way, you will continue to release blockages in a systematic manner. We recommend that you and your partner work in the same way until you can gaze at each other from the lower dantian without any distorted fields getting in the way. Only then should you begin to work in another kanda.

The Mutual Field of Prana

It's not widely known, even among people involved in healing or energy work, that if family members can share enough prana with each other, they will create a field of energy with universal qualities that surrounds them both. This field of energy with universal qualities is called the mutual field of prana.

Once family members have created the mutual field of prana and sustained it for a short time, it will be strong enough to prevent intrusions of energy with individual qualities from interfering with their experience of pleasure, intimacy, and joy. And it will enhance their ability to share energy with universal qualities with one another.

Now, here's the best part: the mutual field of prana will continue to connect partners together—so that they can share pleasure, love, intimacy, and joy even when they're separated from one another by great distances or for long periods of time.

Exercise: The Mutual Field of Prana

To create the mutual field of prana, sit facing your partner, eight feet (two and a half meters) apart. Once you're in position, close your eyes and breathe deeply through your nose for two to three minutes. When you're ready to continue, count backward from five to one and from ten to one. Then assert, *"It's my intent to go to my personal healing space."* Once you've created your personal healing space, bring your awareness to your body, soul, and spirit. Enjoy the process for five minutes. Then assert, *"It's my intent to activate my thirteen chakras in body space."* Once your chakras are active, assert, *"It's my intent to center myself in the chakra fields of my thirteen chakras in body space."* Continue by asserting, *"It's my intent to fill my thirteen chakra fields in body space with prana."* Take a few moments to enjoy the shift. Then assert, *"It's my intent to create a mutual field of prana by radiating prana to my partner from my thirteen chakras in body space."* Don't do anything after that. Just let the energy radiate freely for ten minutes. After ten minutes, count from one to five. When you reach the number five, open your eyes and bring yourself out of the exercise. Repeat the exercise with your partner until you can share prana freely with each other without any distractions or blockages getting in the way.[11]

We taught this exercise to a number of families that we worked with. Simon and Irene were clients who benefited from the experience in a remarkable way. Not only were they able to share more prana with each other and their daughter, but Irene was able to tap into her dormant healing power. She continued to work with us for months afterward and eventually began to use her enhanced empathy and healing power to heal her family, friends, and clients.

EIGHT

The Five Elements and Intimate Relationships

We will begin this chapter by introducing you to Rosalie and her patchwork family. Working through Rosalie's family dynamic was a challenge for us because it involved releasing blockages, projections, and attachments that had poisoned family relationships for at least three generations.

By the time we were finished, we'd worked with Rosalie; her first husband, Cory; their daughter, Sarah, who was six; Rosalie's second husband, Stephen; his ex-wife, Miriam; and their two adolescent daughters, Violet and Amanda, who were eleven and thirteen respectively. Violet and Amanda lived with their mother but spent most weekends and holidays with their grandparents Sam and Bettina, who resented Rosalie and whose resentment and general hostility influenced the family dynamic.

We'll continue by giving you a little additional background. Rosalie married Cory when she was twenty. Within two years, Rosalie gave birth to her first daughter, Sarah. This marriage didn't last because Cory became psychologically violent and he seemed unable to relate in any meaningful way with his daughter. After three tumultuous years, they separated and a year later they divorced.

Cory continued to have contact with Sarah, but after each succeeding visit, Sarah would become increasingly introverted. She wouldn't tell her mother what was wrong. But Rosalie knew something had changed because her daughter lost interest in the things she loved most, including gymnastics and theater.

As a result, Rosalie tried to keep Sarah away from Cory. This was less difficult than she originally imagined since Cory was a workaholic and resented the fact that he had to "entertain Sarah" every other weekend.

When Sarah was five years old, Rosalie met Stephen, a divorced father with two daughters who lived with their mother, Miriam. They married a year later, but Stephen's daughters, Violet and Amanda, never accepted her. In fact, according to Rosalie, "they hated her from the get-go."

To make matters worse, Miriam wanted her ex back, and because of that, she projected her jealousy and resentment into Rosalie's field. She did this intentionally, which made the projections even more disturbing. In her first session with us, we taught Rosalie to stabilize her field by centering herself in her personal healing space (see page 3). Then we taught her to perform the Golden Light Technique (see page 16).

She performed both exercises every day until her following session. In that session, she explained that she had kidney problems and that her bones ached, especially at night. She also told us that she couldn't sense herself and she didn't have the emotional flexibility to participate spontaneously in interactions with other people. These symptoms, as well as her need to control her environment, indicated that she had weak water element and that the dynamics of her patchwork family needed to be addressed in order to heal her.

She went on to explain that she was also concerned that Sarah was often sick and that she was exhibiting behavioral problems in kindergarten. We also learned that Sarah had become excessively dependent on her mother, especially since the divorce. After checking the condition of Sarah's subtle field, we realized that her wood element was weak and needed to be strengthened as well.

We learned much more about Rosalie's patchwork family during the session, but we decided that it was expedient to begin working on the elemental problems first.

Later, we dealt with Stephen's problem with his daughters, Violet and Amanda. He had difficulty sharing his feelings with them and being a trusted ally. In chapter 13, you will learn how Stephen used the techniques of deep family healing to communicate more honestly with his daughters and become a trusted ally whom they could depend on.

The Five Elements

According to the Taoists, the five elements—earth, wood, metal, water, and fire—combine to create the physical and subtle worlds. Like a person's soul vibration and core values, the elements have a significant effect on what a person values, how they interact with family members, and how they feel about themselves.

Sarah seemed to be most disturbed by the family dynamic. In addition to the other symptoms we knew about, including recurrent bladder infections, we observed that she had dark rings around the eyes, clear signs that her water element was weak.

The water element is particularly important to children for two reasons. It influences the development of the subtle field and physical-material body, from birth through puberty. And because it influences the development of a child's personality, it plays a significant part in a child's social interactions with people both inside and outside the home. For these reasons and because of her parents' concern, we began by strengthening Sarah's water element.

If any of the children in your family exhibit the same symptoms as Sarah, we recommend that, like Rosalie, you perform the following exercise every day with your child for at least a month—or until your child has shown significant improvement in these areas.

EXERCISE: Strengthening the Water Element

In order to strengthen Sarah's water element, we taught Rosalie to fill the associated organs in her daughter's body with blue prana and to chant the sound *fff* during the exercise. The organs associated with the water element include the ears, teeth, kidneys, bladder, and bones—especially the spine.

After you've filled these organs with blue prana, you will keep your attention focused on them while you chant *fff* for ten minutes.

To begin the exercise, find a comfortable position with your back straight close to your child. Close your eyes and breathe deeply through your nose for two to three minutes. Then count backward from five to one and from ten to one. Continue by asserting, *"It's my intent to go to my personal healing space."* Then bring your awareness to your body, soul, and spirit. Enjoy your healing space for five minutes. Then assert, *"It's my intent to fill…* (child's name)*'s ears, bones, spine, teeth, kidneys, and bladder with blue prana."* Enjoy the process for another five minutes. Then chant *fff* with your child for ten minutes more while you stay focused on the same organs. After you finished chanting with your child, count from one to five. When you reach the number five, open your eyes and bring yourself out of the exercise. Repeat the exercise regularly until the organs associated with the element are once again functioning healthfully.

Once Rosalie began to see tangible improvements in Sarah's condition, she began working on her water element, which also needed to be strengthened. And within weeks she achieved the same positive results as Sarah.

Determining Which Elements are Weak

Like Rosalie and Sarah, most people have at least one weak element that interferes with their well-being and their family relationships.

Taoist adepts have provided us with a number of markers that indicate whether one or more of your elements have been weakened over time. In the following text, we've listed the most common markers. By checking them against your present condition, you will be able to determine if one of your elements is weak and needs to be strengthened.

In most cases, two or more markers will indicate that you have a weak element. Like Rosalie and Sarah, once you've determined which of your elements are weak, you can strengthen them by practicing the same exercise they did or one of the variations listed below. The first element we will look at is metal.

Weak Metal: On the physical-material level, respiratory ailments and colon problems are signs of a weak metal element. Thyroid problems and all problems affecting the breath also serve as markers. Dry skin and excessive sweating as well diarrhea and weight problems have been commonly associated with a weak metal element.

On the non-physical level, a weak metal element will disrupt self-esteem, mental stability, and deductive and inductive reasoning. It will disrupt self-confidence as well as the ability to make life-affirming decisions.

Sadness and pain are the emotions associated with a weak metal element, as is excessive crying.

If your metal element is weak, you will have difficulty with interpersonal issues that involve attachment, space, and distance. Excessive sensitivity and dependence as well as a lack of discipline are all associated with weak metal. So are depression and a lack of motivation. Another marker which is closely related to a weak metal element is attachment to the past—and the yearning for a relationship that is no longer possible.

Weak Water: On the physical-material level, a weak water element can create kidney problems, recurrent bladder infections, hearing problems and tinnitus. Weak and painful joints and bones, knee problems, and lower back pain can indicate a weak water element. Premature hair loss and dental problems are also associated with weak water—so are persistent dark rings around the eyes.

On the non-physical level, a weak water element can create fear and anxiety as well as panic attacks, instability, and a lack of stick-to-it-iveness. People with a weak water element are also prone to addiction. A lack of courage and perseverance, and an inability to let go of attachments, are signs of a weak water element. So is the tendency to give away personal responsibility and become dependent on others.

Weak Fire: On the physical-material level, a weak fire element can cause high blood pressure and mechanical problems associated with the heart. Blood problems, anemia, diarrhea, and inflammation of the small intestine as well as other organs and tissues of the digestive tract are also markers. So is burnout.

People with a weak fire element have a need to be accepted. They have difficulty giving or receiving love and/or experiencing sexual joy. Superficial relationships devoid of real intimacy are therefore markers of a weak fire element. So are lethargy and a lack of perseverance. Persistent annoyance and irritation as well as problems completing projects or finishing projects on time also indicate a weak fire element.

Weak Earth: Problems with the mouth, lips, spleen, pancreas, thymus gland, stomach, lymphatic system, and the joints, especially the hip joints, indicate a weak earth element. Feelings of heaviness in the arms and legs as well as swelling and cellulite also serve as markers. Metabolic problems, abdominal bloating, pain, and hormonal imbalances as well as varicose veins can also indicate a weak earth element.

Excessive worry, depression, and information overload are also markers—so is an obsession with money and security. People whose earth element is weak can become dependent and needy. They can binge on alcohol, drugs, and food. Some may eat sweets to excess and, as a result, experience excessive weight gain. In extreme cases, a person with a weak earth element can feel that they have a hole inside themselves that can't be filled.

Weak Wood is associated with liver and gall bladder ailments. Problems with the shoulders, eyes, ligaments, and the muscles of the body as well as dizziness and headaches are all associated with a weak wood element. Excessive menstrual pain in women can also serve as a marker.

The emotions associated with weak wood are anger and rage. If neither of these emotions can be released in a healthy way, then a person can become rigid and closed to new ideas. Creativity can be disrupted when the wood element is weak. Self-destructive feelings and guilt are clear signs that the wood element has been weakened. So is the inability to set clear goals and achieve them.

Strengthening Weak Elements

Like Rosalie and Sarah, you can strengthen a weak element by filling the organs associated with it with prana in the appropriate color—and by chanting the appropriate sound during the exercise. This makes strengthening a weak element easy because every element is associated with both a specific color and sound that matches its mean frequency. The organs, colors, and tones associated with the elements are included in the list below.

Metal: The organs associated with metal include the nose, sinuses, bronchial system, lungs, diaphragm, colon, and skin. The color associated with metal is white, the sound *sss.*

Water: The organs associated with the water element include the kidneys, bones, bladder, marrow, teeth, hair, and ears. The color associated with water is dark blue, the sound *fff.*

Fire: The organs associated with fire include the heart, blood, small intestine, and the other organs and tissues of the digestive tract. The color associated with fire is red, the sound *hhaa.*

Earth: The organs associated with earth include the stomach, spleen, and pancreas. The color associated with earth is yellow, the sound *hyyu.*

Wood: The organs associated with wood include the liver, gall bladder, shoulders, eyes, ligaments, and the muscles of the body. The color associated with wood is green, the sound *schh.*

If you've determined that one of your elements or one of the elements of a family member is weak after studying the markers, then, like Rosalie and Sarah, you can use the last exercise and/or one of its variations to strengthen it.

Kidney Jing

After Rosalie finished strengthening the appropriate elements for both herself and her daughter, we taught her to strengthen their kidney jing. Kidney jing, the essence of chi, is closely related to kidney chi.

We also taught a young couple from New York, Hanna and Barry, to strengthen their kidney jing. Hanna consulted us in the winter of 2014 when she was twenty-nine years old. In her first session with us, she complained that her two-year-old daughter, Amy, was constantly sick and her husband, Barry, who was thirty-four, refused to have sex with her because he felt exhausted afterward. To make matters worse, Barry had developed an erectile dysfunction—and he blamed her for the problem. Although blame only served to complicate the issues involved, we quickly discerned that the problem was rooted in Hanna's and Barry's lack of kidney jing.

Hanna's kidney jing was being disrupted by Monica, a disgruntled colleague, who had been stealing from her company and who blamed Hanna for her dismissal. Without enough kidney jing to support her sexual relationship with her husband, Hanna had inadvertently begun to draw energy from Barry's and Amy's energy fields. This had dire effects on both their personal well-being and their ability to participate in healthy family relationships, because the kidneys are resevoirs of jing. It also interfered with the couple's goal of having a second child.

Before you learn to strengthen your kidney jing, like Hanna and Barry did, you need to know more about how jing influences your well-being and family relationships. Jing is essence. Like the life force, it connects everything that lives and breathes. Although it pervades the internal and external environment of all living things—and the universe as a whole—for the sake of convenience, we can say that it has three locations that interact with one another. There is eternal jing, which permeates the universe and interacts with your subtle field on both the macrocosmic and microcosmic levels; there is external jing, which surrounds you and radiates through your field, and there is internal jing, which is a field of jing located by your perineum. The internal field is connected to the kidneys and the eight exceptional meridians—including the two most important meridians, the governor and conceptual.

The Importance of the Kidneys

There are two types of jing, ancestral jing and acquired jing. Both are stored in the kidneys as well as the exceptional meridians. There are eight exceptional meridians including the conceptual, governor, and thorax meridians, which distribute jing throughout the subtle field and physical-material body.

The function of jing is to promote growth, development, and reproduction. Ancestral jing comes from one's parents and determines basic constitution; it cannot be altered, but it can be positively influenced by acquired jing. The sources of acquired jing include the eternal field of jing and foods such as seeds, nuts (particularly walnuts), beans and peas, mussels, oatmeal, dried fruit, hot soups, and cooked root vegetables.

Life-affirming relationships and environments are also important sources of acquired jing. The interaction of ancestral jing and acquired jing produces kidney jing.

When kidney jing has been disrupted on either the energetic or physical-material level, you can experience a lack of vitality and a disruption of your sexuality. An inability to feel and/or express your natural feelings and sensations is another common symptom. You can also suffer from problems with your bones, teeth, joints, ears, and urinary tract.

When you lack kidney jing, pervasive fear and/or anxiety can begin to interfere with your relationships. Your ability to resist negative influences can also be weakened, which can make you more susceptible to energetic and physical traumas.

Additional symptoms that indicate weak kidney jing include cold extremities, heat waves or flashes, disk problems, bone loss, back pain, recurrent bladder infections, and prostate problems. Hair loss, gum inflammation, tinnitus, hearing issues, and menstrual problems are also associated with weak kidney jing.

In children, a lack of kidney jing can cause developmental problems on both the physical and mental levels. Because of its proximity to the lower dantian and because it's so closely associated to the life force, the Chinese refer to the kidneys as the "Origin of Life."

It's possible to strengthen acquired jing by eating the foods we mentioned above—and by spending time in harmonious environments with people whose outlook is life-affirming. You can also strengthen kidney jing by strengthening your relationship to the three fields of jing.

If you've determined that your kidney jing is weak from what you've just learned, we recommend that you perform the Jing Recognition Technique. This exercise will provide you a direct experience of jing in its three forms: eternal jing, which is the source of all jing in the universe and can be compared to the life force; external jing, which surrounds you and creates a stable environment for all energetic interactions in your subtle field and physical-material body; and internal jing, which is located by the perineum. It supplies the kidneys with jing and governs the general distribution of universal energy throughout your body and soul.

All three fields of jing can be disrupted by distorted fields of energy. In the following exercise, you will use your intent to experience jing in all three forms.

We recommend that you perform this exercise in a natural setting without the interference of other people and electronic devices. By doing that, it's possible to experience a sense of oneness with the ecology of life on the physical-material and subtle levels.

EXERCISE: The Jing Recognition Technique

To begin the exercise, find a comfortable position with your back straight. Close your eyes and breathe deeply through your nose for two to three minutes. Then count backward from five to one and from ten to one. Continue by asserting, *"It's my intent to go to my personal healing space."* Then bring your awareness to your body, soul, and spirit. Enjoy your healing space for five minutes. Then assert, *"It's my intent to experience the eternal field of jing."* Take five minutes to enjoy the experience. Then assert, *"It's my intent to experience my external field of jing."* Continue to enjoy it for five minutes. Then assert, *"It's my intent to experience my internal field of jing."* After you've experienced your internal field of jing for five minutes, count from one to five. When you reach the number five, open your eyes and bring yourself out of the meditation.

It's not unusual to experience a pervasive buzz in your body after you've performed the exercise. This indicates that you've begun to enhance your level of vitality.

The next exercise is the Jing Enhancement Technique. By performing it after you've experienced your three fields of jing, you will enhance the amount of acquired jing you have in your kidneys.

EXERCISE: The Jing Enhancement Technique

To begin the exercise, find a comfortable position with your back straight. Close your eyes and breathe deeply through your nose for two to three minutes. Then count backward from five to one and from ten to one. Continue by asserting, *"It's my intent to go to my personal healing space."* Then bring your awareness to your body, soul, and spirit. Enjoy your healing space for five minutes. Then assert, *"It's my intent to experience my eternal, external, and internal fields of jing."* Take five minutes to enjoy the shift. Then assert, *"It's my intent to enhance the flow of jing from the eternal field of jing into my external field of jing."* Take five minutes to enjoy the process. Then assert, *"It's my intent to enhance the flow of jing from my external field of jing into my internal field of jing and from there into my kidneys."* Take another ten minutes to enjoy the process. Then bring yourself out of the exercise by counting from one to five. When you reach the number five, open your eyes. You will feel wide awake, perfectly relaxed, and better than you did before.

The next issue we dealt with was the influence of Miriam's jealousy, which she had been projecting at Rosalie and Stephen in the form of distorted fields of energy.

We contacted Miriam, but she was intransigent and refused to have anything to do with the healing process. In order to protect Rosalie and Stephen from the constant intrusion of Miriam's projections, we taught them to strengthen their Wei chi (Guardian Chi). We did that by teaching them to perform the Jing Restoration Technique, which you will find in the following text.

But first, a few words of explanation. There are several meridians within the subtle field that are tasked with protecting the subtle field from intrusions of distorted energy. They do this by absorbing chi from nearby meridians and jing from the kidneys. Then they use the energy and its essence to create a shield that blocks the intrusion of distorted energy ("evil chi"). They are known as exceptional meridians and they include:

1. The Governor meridian (Du Mai). It originates at the perineum and ascends through the spine into the crown of the head where it terminates.

2. The Conceptual meridian (Ren Mai). It originates at the front of the seventh chakra gate and descends down the front of the body to the first chakra at the perineum.

3. The Thrusting Vessel (Chong Mai). It originates at the perineum and moves up to the pubic bone. It continues through the abdomen into the chest and from there into the face.

4. Girdle Meridian (Dai Mai). Its course takes it around the waist in the region of the lower dantian.

5. Yang Heel Vessel (Yangchiao Mai). It originates at the heel of the left foot and moves upward along the left side of the body to the eye. From there it traverses the head terminating on the right side of the back of the head.

6. Yin Heel Vessel (Yinchiao Mai). It originates at the heel of the right foot and moves upward along the right side of the body to the eye. From there it traverses the head terminating at the left side of the back of the head.

7. Yang Linking Vessel (Yangwei Mai). It originates at the heel of the left foot. It continues up the inside of the left leg through the trunk until it reaches the throat. From there it moves up the

center of the neck to the top of the head. It completes its journey at the point where the back of the neck meets the skull.

8. Yin Linking Vessel (Yinwei Mai). It originates at the heel of the right foot. It continues up the inside of the right leg through the trunk until it reaches the throat. From there it moves up the center of the neck to the top of the head. It completes its journey at the point where the back of the neck meets the skull (see figure 14: The Eight Exceptional Meridians, page 127–130).

By strengthening the exceptional meridians and the flow of kidney chi (jing) through them, it's possible to protect the most vulnerable parts of the subtle field—the abdomen, thorax, and back—from projections of distorted energy. In Rosalie's case, this was essential since Miriam's projections interfered with the functions of both her third chakra and the movement of jing through her microcosmic circuit.

Exercise: The Jing Restoration Technique

To begin the exercise, find a comfortable position with your back straight. Close your eyes and breathe deeply through your nose for two to three minutes. Then count backward from five to one and from ten to one. Continue by asserting, *"It's my intent to go to my personal healing space."* Then bring your awareness to your body, soul, and spirit. Enjoy your healing space for five minutes. Then assert, *"It's my intent to center myself in my field of eternal jing."* Enjoy it for two to three minutes. Then assert, *"It's my intent that jing from my eternal field of jing flows into my external field of jing and fills it."* Take another five minutes to enjoy the process. Then assert, *"It's my intent that that jing from my external field of jing flows into my internal field of jing and from there into my kidneys and exceptional meridians."* Take another ten minutes to experience the changes the extra jing brings to your body, soul, and spirit. Then count from one to five. When you reach the number five, open your eyes and bring yourself out of the exercise.

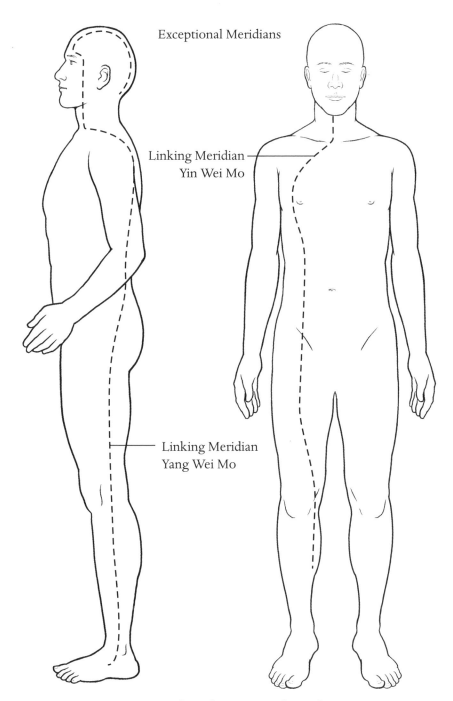

Exceptional Meridians

Linking Meridian
Yin Wei Mo

Linking Meridian
Yang Wei Mo

Figure 14: The Eight Exceptional Meridians

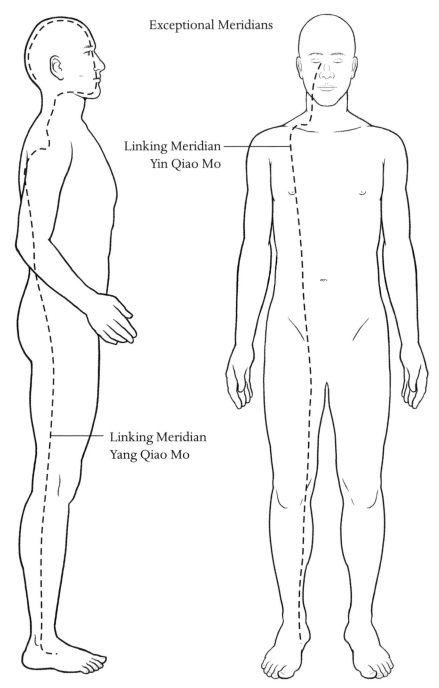

Exceptional Meridians

Linking Meridian
Yin Qiao Mo

Linking Meridian
Yang Qiao Mo

Figure 14A: The Eight Exceptional Meridians (continued)

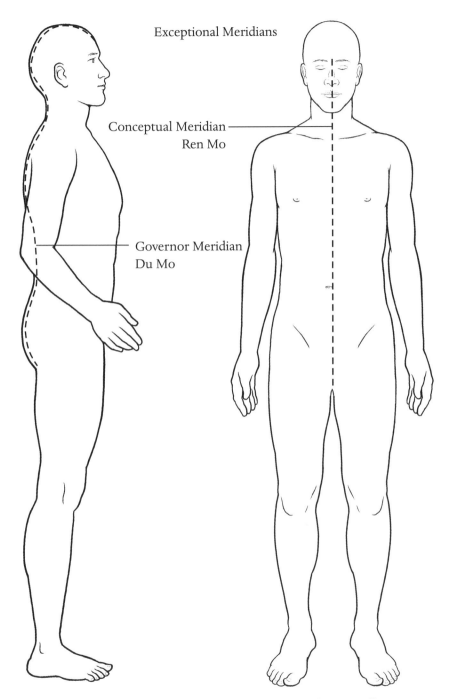

Figure 14B: The Eight Exceptional Meridians (continued)

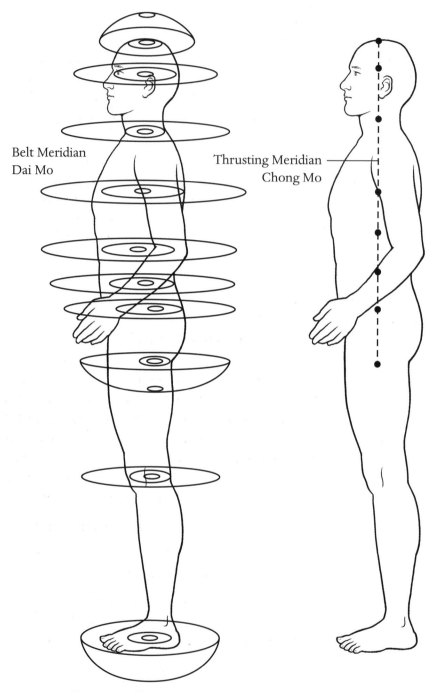

Belt Meridian
Dai Mo

Thrusting Meridian
Chong Mo

Figure 14C: The Eight Exceptional Meridians (continued)

Hanna and Barry performed the exercises for several months. Although they experienced a gradual improvement, the exercises did not heal the family dynamic completely. To complete the process, we taught them to perform the Boundary Safety Net because Monica, whom Hanna testified against, continued to project at her.

NINE

Overcoming Self-Limiting Patterns

Although there is a great deal that you can do to heal your family relationships, it's often what you stop doing that has the most salutary effect on them. In this chapter, we've included a list of five destructive patterns that you must overcome in order to restore your family relationships to a state of radiant good health.

The five patterns are listed below, along with a description of their effects on you and your family relationships. Following each pattern, you will find a simple exercise or series of exercises that have been used successfully by other families to overcome the pattern permanently. If you've been trapped by any of the patterns in our list, practice the exercises we've provided until the pattern no longer disturbs you or interferes with your relationships.

Pattern 1: Withholding

People who are withholding are unable to express themselves, communicate, or share their feelings and emotions freely with other people including their family members. This makes sharing pleasure, love, intimacy, and joy difficult.

It's the fear of confronting distorted energy fields and/or the inability to radiate prana and jing freely that sustains the pattern of withholding and prevents most people from overcoming it.

This pattern continued to influence Andrew's relationship to his two sons Mark and Luke and was instrumental in alienating them from him. It also was part of the group of patterns that had prevented Alan from establishing a healthy relationship with his stepson Dennis.

There are many dynamics created by traditional and non-traditional families that can block an adult's feelings and emotions and the energy that supports them. The adult child may have had parents who created an environment of fear and/or judgment. This was the case with Andrew's patchwork family; the adult child may have had a step-parent that withheld affection or rejected the child outright. Another possibility is that siblings competed with the adult child for attention. There are too many possibilities to list all of them here. The important point is that, if you're stuck in a pattern of withholding, it's essential to get the blocked energy and jing flowing again.

A successful businessman named Henry, who lived in Seattle, was at a loss to explain why he was unable to sustain a relationship with a woman for more than a few months. He was forty-two when he consulted us—attractive and a self-starter who'd developed a software program that made him rich. Although he complained that none of the women he met were his type, we quickly recognized that the problem stemmed from his self-importance and the withholding pattern that he believed had helped him succeed in business.

What he didn't realize was that both patterns originated in the foster home where he was raised—and where he was considered to be an interloper by his older foster brother and withholding foster father. Unfortunately, like many successful people, he believed that the same personality traits that had helped him succeed in business would help him succeed in his personal relationships. In fact, rather than ingratiate him with women he dated, those traits did the opposite. They turned them off. In the end, he did find a compatible partner—but only after he'd overcome the pattern of withholding and had strengthened his character.

Solution: to overcome their withholding pattern, Andrew and Henry used the Jing Enhancement Technique to enhance their supply of acquired jing and the Granti Cleansing Technique to release distorted fields of energy that prevented jing from being distributed in a balanced way through their subtle fields.

To perform the Jing Enhancement Technique, see page 124. Once you've performed the technique every day for a week, perform the Granti Cleansing

Technique along with it every day for at least two more weeks or until with-holding is no longer an issue for you.

EXERCISE: The Granti Cleansing Technique

Grantis are fields of distorted energy that can interfere with the func-tions of the kidneys, kandas, and the exceptional meridians. Because they can interfere with the functions of these vital organs, they can block the transfer of chi from chakra fields and kandas to the micro-cosmic circuit and their subsidiary meridians. They can also interfere with the transfer of jing from the internal field of jing to the kidneys, the exceptional meridians, and the physical-material body. Unlike kandas or chakra fields, grantis are concentrations of distorted energy that accumulate near the kandas. The larger the grantis become, the more negative their effect will be. There are three grantis that can in-terfere directly with the microcosmic circuit and the kidneys.

The lower granti is located just behind the first chakra gate in the region of the first kanda. The middle granti is located just behind the fourth chakra gate, in the region of the second kanda. And the upper granti is located just behind the sixth chakra gate behind the head, in the region of the third kanda (see figure 15: The Three Grantis, page 137).

To begin the exercise, find a comfortable position with your back straight. Then breathe deeply through your nose for two to three min-utes. Continue by asserting, *"It's my intent to go to my personal healing space."* Then bring your awareness to your body, soul, and spirit. Enjoy your healing space for five minutes. Then assert, *"It's my intent to locate my lower granti."* Once you've located the granti, observe its condition with your appropriate organs of perception, paying particular attention to its size and density. After you're satisfied that you have seen and/or sensed its condition, assert, *"It's my intent to locate the most distorted field of energy in my lower granti."* Once you can sense or see the dis-torted field, which will look darker and feel heavier than the surround-ing energy, assert, *"It's my intent to surround the distorted field of energy I have in mind with a prana box."* Once you can see and/or sense the box, assert, *"It's my intent to fill the prana box with prana and to release the distorted field of energy within it.*" Don't do anything after that. Prana will fill the box you've created and release the distorted field of energy automatically. Continue to enjoy the process for five minutes more. Then count from one to five. When you reach the number five, open your eyes and bring yourself out of the meditation.

Some of you may experience a sense of relief and well-being after prana fills the box. That indicates that the distorted field within the box has been released and prana has filled the vacated space. Continue to perform the exercise regularly, always releasing the most distorted field that remains, until all the distorted fields blocking your kidneys and your ability to express yourself freely have been released.

Pattern 2: Narcissism

Narcissism is more than a distorted form of self-love. It's a form of self-involvement that compels the narcissistic person to put themselves at the center of all interpersonal interactions including interactions with their friends and family members. A person can get stuck in a pattern of narcissism when their ego has usurped the role of their authentic mind or their I-field has been engorged by fields of distorted consciousness. In either case, the subject's authentic identity and ability to engage in honest and authentic relationships will be disrupted.

Like the grantis, neither the ego nor the I-field are authentic organs of the subtle field. Both are created by concentrations of energy with individual qualities. The ego is located in the front of body space in the region of the fourth chakra. The stronger and more disruptive the ego has become, the larger and denser it will be.

The I-field is dispersed throughout the subtle field. In extreme cases, when the ego and I-field have usurped the functions of the authentic mind, they can combine with the grantis and other distorted fields to form an inauthentic identity.

Before we move on, it's important to note that everyone has an authentic identity. Yoga divides a person's authentic identity into two parts, an individual identity and a universal identity. In Sanskrit, the sacred language of India, individual identity is known as *jivamatman*, and universal identity is known as *paramatman*.

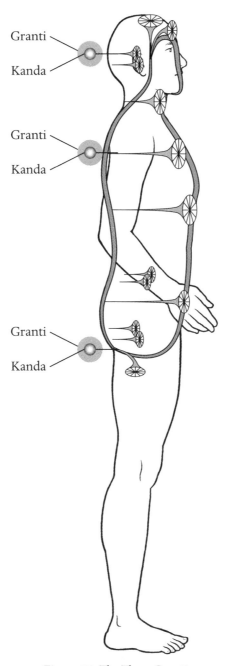

Granti

Kanda

Granti

Kanda

Granti

Kanda

Figure 15: The Three Grantis

The strength of a person's individual identity will determine whether they will have the resources to successfully participate in a long-term relationship. The strength of their universal identity will determine whether they will be able to achieve and sustain intimacy with a family member in all situations.

If the pattern of narcissism disrupts your individual identity, interferes with your authentic feelings and emotions, and prevents you from having the resources to participate in a long-term relationship, the foundation is in the ego.

If the pattern disrupts your universal identity, blocks your awareness and perception, and makes it difficult for you to achieve or sustain intimacy, then the problem has its foundation in the I-field. If you are unable to do either, then the problem is rooted in both the ego and the I-field.

The foundation of Andrew's narcissism was distorted I-fields that his father had projected at him and to which he had become attached. At first, he had a problem recognizing this because the very idea elicited fear. To overcome his fear, we taught him to perform the Fearless Mudra to calm his mind and to facilitate his process of reflection (see figure 18: The Fearless Mudra, page 164). Then we asked him to hold a note in each of his hands while he reflected on the pattern.

The note in his right hand stated, "It's my desire to experience the truth about my pattern of narcissism." The note in his left hand stated, "It's my will to know what supports my pattern of narcissism." He performed this ritual every day for two weeks and discovered that when he tried to center himself in his chest or abdomen, he was blocked. He explained, "When I try to center myself, I feel like there is a hole in my center, and when I try to feel what is in the hole, my awareness is forcibly pushed outside my body space."

From what he told us, we recognized that the problem was caused by I-fields which had taken control over the front of his body and had left virtually no room for paramatman to emerge and to radiate its universal qualities freely.

Solution: Overcoming a pattern of narcissism is a process that will involve healing yourself as well as healing your family relationships. In the first part of the process, you must determine the root cause of the problem.

If the root cause of the problem lies in both the ego and I-field, you will begin by locating and releasing the most distorted field in the ego using the Bliss Box Technique. When all the offending fields in the ego have been released you will shift your attention to the your I-field and release the offending fields, beginning with the most distorted field, until all the distorted fields supporting the pattern have been released.

In the next part of the process, you will fill your three fields of empathy with bliss every day for a week. We recommend that you do that as soon as you've released the distorted fields that supported the pattern.

EXERCISE: Cleansing the Ego
or I-Field with the Bliss Box

To begin the exercise, find a comfortable position with your back straight. Then breathe deeply through your nose for two to three minutes. Use the Orgasmic Bliss Mudra to bring bliss into your conscious awareness (see figure 9: The Orgasmic Bliss Mudra, page 70).

Hold the mudra for five minutes. If the offending fields are in the ego, then assert, *"It's my intent to experience the most distorted field in my ego that supports my pattern of narcissism."* If the offending field is in the I-field, then substitute I-field for ego. Once you can sense or see the distorted field, which will look darker than the surrounding fields, assert, *"It's my intent to surround the distorted field I have in mind with a bliss box."* Once you can sense and/or see the bliss box, assert, *"It's my intent to fill the bliss box with bliss and to release the distorted field within it."* Don't do anything after that. Bliss will fill the box you've created and release the distorted field automatically. Continue to enjoy the process for ten minutes more. Then count from one to five. When you reach the number five, release the bliss mudra. Then open your eyes and bring yourself out of the exercise. Continue to perform the same exercise on the most distorted field that remains in your ego or I-field until all the distorted fields that support the pattern have been released.

Some of you may experience a sense of relief and well-being when bliss fills the box. That indicates that the distorted field within the box has been released and bliss has filled the vacated space.

Exercise: Filling the Fields of Empathy with Bliss

To begin this exercise, find a comfortable position with your back straight. Then close your eyes and breathe deeply through your nose for two to three minutes. To continue, count backward from five to one and from ten to one. Then perform the Orgasmic Bliss Mudra (see figure 9: The Orgasmic Bliss Mudra, page 70). Continue to hold the mudra while you assert, *"It's my intent to center myself in my three fields of empathy."* Continue by asserting, *"It's my intent to turn my appropriate organs of perception inward on the level of my three fields of empathy."* Take a moment to enjoy the shift. Then assert, *"It's my intent to fill my three fields of empathy with bliss."* Take about fifteen minutes to fill your three fields of empathy with bliss. Then count from one to five. When you reach the number five, release the Orgasmic Bliss Mudra, open your eyes, and bring yourself out of the exercise. Continue to perform the exercise every day for seven consecutive days.

Pattern 3: Dependency

Dependent people have a distorted view of love and intimacy. Instead of nourishing their relationships with prana, jing, and pure consciousness, they weaken their relationships by projecting fields of distorted energy at their relationship partners. They do that in order to hold on to a person they consider significant or to create a relationship that makes them feel comfortable, even if their comfort comes at the expense of someone else.

Solution: Since dependency is related to both a lack of self-esteem and a lack of personal power, to overcome the pattern, you will perform three exercises. For the first two weeks of the process, you will perform the Self-Esteem Mudra. Starting in the third week, you will replace the Self-Esteem Mudra with the Dantian Vitality Technique and the Microcosmic Circuit Meditation. We recommend that you continue to practice both exercises every day for at least a month—or until dependency has become a thing of the past.

EXERCISE: The Self-Esteem Mudra

To perform the Self-Esteem Mudra, sit in a comfortable position with your back straight. Breathe deeply through your nose for two to three minutes. Then form a cup with your hands. Once you've formed the cup, place the sides of your thumbs together and your left index fingers—from the tip to the first joint—over the tip of the right index finger as far as the first joint. Do the same with your middle fingers. Then put the tips of your ring fingers and the tips of your pinky fingers together. Press your tongue up against the roof of your mouth and slide it back until the roof becomes soft. Then put the soles of your feet together. Hold the mudra for ten minutes while you breathe in and out from your solar plexus.

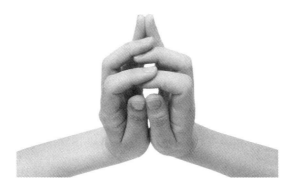

Figure 16: The Self-Esteem Mudra

EXERCISE: Dantian Vitality Technique

To begin the exercise, find a comfortable position with your back straight. Then close your eyes and breathe deeply through your nose for two to three minutes. Continue by asserting, *"It's my intent to go to my personal healing space."* Then bring your awareness to your body, soul, and spirit. Enjoy your healing space for five minutes. Then assert, *"It's my intent to center myself in my lower dantian."* Once you're centered, assert, *"It's my intent to fill my lower dantian with chi and jing."* Take five minutes to enjoy the process. Then remove your mental attention from your lower dantian and assert, *"It's my intent to center myself in my middle dantian."* Once you're centered, assert, *"It's my intent to fill my middle dantian with chi and jing."* Take five minutes to enjoy the process. Then remove your mental attention from your middle dantian and assert, *"It's my intent to center myself in my upper dantian."* Once you're centered, assert, *"It's my intent to fill my upper dantian with chi and jing."* Continue to enjoy the process for ten minutes more. Then count from one to five. When you reach the number five, open your eyes and bring yourself out of the exercise.

Practice the Dantian Vitality Technique every day for a week along with the following exercise.

EXERCISE: The Microcosmic Circuit Meditation

To perform the Microcosmic Circuit Meditation, see page 108.

Perform the Microcosmic Circuit Meditation along with the Dantian Vitality Technique for at least a month more or until the pattern of dependency no longer influences your relationships.

Pattern 4: Control

People who need to control their environment (and other people) cannot express their feelings or emotions freely or experience unconditional joy because they lack space within themselves on the subtle levels of energy and consciousness. The problem can be caused by several interlocking patterns that prevent an adult from accepting things without having to modify their environment.

There are two issues that must be addressed in order to heal this pattern and the relationship problems that it creates. The first issue is the lack of space in the subtle field created by blockages in the kidneys. These blockages can prevent jing emerging from the internal field of jing from radiating into the kidneys and exceptional meridians. Without enough jing, a person will be trapped within a severely limited comfort zone without the ability to express themselves freely.

The second issue is the disruption of the family dynamic. Family members will suffer from the projections of the controlling family member because the controlling family member will be compelled to project distorted energy into the family field in an effort to control the family environment. Projections such as these will interfere with the well-being of family members and will eventually disrupt family relationships.

We faced this situation when we worked with Hanna. To restore the space she needed on the subtle levels, we helped her to enhance her kidney jing. Once her kidney jing was restored to a healthy level, we began to heal the family dynamic by having Hanna locate and release the controlling fields she had projected at her husband and children.

Solution: To overcome Hanna's need to control, we had her use the Prana Box Technique to release blockages in her kidneys. Then she filled them with internal jing. By the time she'd finished, she had more space to express her feelings and authentic emotions freely and to feel unconditional joy once again. We also had her use the prana box to release the controlling waves she'd projected at her husband and children. After Hanna overcame her pattern of control, we taught her along with Barry to perform the Boundary Safety Net, which you will learn to perform in chapter 17.

EXERCISE: Kidney Chi Restoration Technique

To begin the exercise, find a comfortable position with your back straight. Then close your eyes and breathe deeply through your nose for two to three minutes. Continue by asserting, *"It's my intent to go to my personal healing space."* Then bring your awareness to your body, soul, and spirit. Enjoy your healing space for five minutes. Then assert, *"It's my intent to surround my right kidney with a prana box."* As soon as you can see and/or feel the prana box, assert, *"It's my intent to fill the prana box with prana and release all the distorted fields within it."* Since the prana that fills the box will be releasing several fields at once, give the process some time to be completed (see the following text). Once you feel that the blockages have been released, assert, *"It's my intent to surround my left kidney with a prana box."* As soon as you can see and/or feel the prana box, assert, *"It's my intent to fill the prana box with prana and release all the distorted fields within it."* After giving the process enough time to finish, assert, *"It's my intent to fill my kidneys and the exceptional meridians with jing from my internal jing field."* By filling your kidneys and exceptional meridians with internal jing, you will not only enhance the amount of jing you have available but enhance its ability to flow freely through your subtle field.

Enjoy the process for ten minutes more. Then count from one to five. When you reach the number five, open your eyes and bring yourself out of the exercise. We recommend that you practice the exercise every day for two weeks—or until the pattern of control no longer disturbs you or your relationships.

Once you're confident that prana has replaced the blockages you've released, you must locate the controlling waves that you projected at your family members and release them. To do that, you will use the Visual Screen Technique and the Prana Box Technique.

Controlling waves are waves of energy with individual qualities. In most cases, they're projected by someone who seeks to control their environment and/or change an aspect of another person's behavior and/or personality.

Controlling waves are normally wedge-shaped when they emerge from the perpetrator's energy field. However, once the controlling wave has entered a family member's energy field, it will quickly expand until it fills a large portion of it.

Whenever someone projects an attitude, thought, emotion, feeling, or inauthentic desire at a family member, they can project a controlling wave.

In most cases, the controlling wave will remain intact as long as it serves the perpetrator's purpose, which can be as simple as holding on to someone, even if the desire or need for relationship isn't reciprocated. You can use the following exercise to locate and release a controlling wave that you or someone in your family has projected at another family member. Always begin by releasing the most disruptive controlling wave and continue until all of the controlling waves have been released.

EXERCISE: Releasing Controlling Waves

To begin the exercise, choose a family member who you believe has been affected by your need to control. Then find a comfortable position with your back straight. Close your eyes and breathe deeply through your nose for two to three minutes. Then count backward from five to one and from ten to one. Continue by asserting, *"It's my intent to go to my personal healing space."* Then bring your awareness to your body, soul, and spirit. Enjoy your healing space for five minutes. Then assert, *"It's my intent to create a white screen eight feet* (two and a half meters) *in front of me."* Once the visual screen has materialized, assert, *"It's my intent to visualize* (name of family member) *on the screen."* Immediately, you will see their image appear on the screen in a size to fit comfortably. Observe it for about two to three minutes; then assert, *"It's my intent to locate the most distorted controlling wave that I projected at* (family member's name)*."* Observe it for a moment. Then assert, *"It's my intent to surround the controlling wave I have in mind with a prana box."* Once the box appears, assert, *"It's my intent to fill the prana box with prana and release the controlling wave within it."* Don't do anything else. The prana in the box will release the controlling wave automatically. After the controlling wave has been released, release the image you created and the visual screen. Then count from one to five. When you reach the number five, open your eyes and bring yourself out of the exercise.

Some of you may experience a sense of relief and well-being when prana fills the box. That indicates that the controlling wave within the box has been released and prana has filled the vacated space.

We recommend that you continue to perform the same exercise on the most distorted controlling wave that remains until all of the controlling waves that you projected at a family member have been released.

Pattern 5: Chaos

A pattern of chaos can be created if your field of chaos has become overloaded with destabilizing fields of energy and consciousness. The pattern can be aggravated further by the projection of distorted energy or consciousness into a specific area of your subtle field by someone who has focused their minds on you—or consistently disapproves of you and what you are doing.

The field of chaos serves as a collection center, where subtle fields that contribute to chaos are gathered. Once enough of these fields have accumulated, they will interfere with your ability to participate in healthy family relationships by disrupting the functions of your authentic mind.

If you consistently project chaos into your relationships because you're undependable, jealous, don't know what you want, can't finish anything you start, or can't relax or feel empathy for other people, then you are trapped in chaotic fields of energy and/or consciousness.

Solution: If you've determined that you suffer from a pattern of chaos, you can overcome it by performing an exercise we developed from a guiding principle of the Bhagavad Gita. The Gita, a revered Yogic text, teaches that enlightenment can only be achieved when the field of knowledge (the physical and non-physical universe), the knower (your authentic mind), and knowledge (universal energy and consciousness) become one.

People who are chaotic and project subtle fields of chaos at other people are trapped in the field of knowledge (the physical and non-physical universe) without access to the knower (the authentic mind) and knowledge (universal energy and consciousness). To liberate yourself from chaos, you will center yourself in field of the knower first. Then you will center yourself in the field of knowledge—both of which will emerge as large fields within your subtle field. Once you've centered yourself in each field, you will fill them with prana and bliss. If you fill both fields with prana and bliss every day for a month, chaos will diminish and you will feel more stable and secure in your subtle field.

Our work with Jose and Monica illustrates how chaos can disrupt an otherwise healthy relationship. Jose and Monica consulted us in 2012. Jose had been a surfer for most of his life. But in his early forties, he'd developed severe arthritis in his ankles and shoulders, which made it impossible for him to continue surfing. Surfing had always had a soothing effect on Jose's otherwise active mind. It had calmed his nerves and shielded him from the worst effects of his relationship with his alcoholic father. Without his sport, which he'd practiced since he was a child, his thinking became overwhelmingly negative and chaotic. This disrupted his business, a surf shop, which he'd owned for more than twenty years. And it had begun to undermine his relationship to Monica, who—because of his chaotic condition—had started an affair with a local surfer-turned-businessman.

In order to overcome the pattern of chaos, we had Jose perform the Stability Restoration Technique in the following text. We recommend that you try it if you suffer from a pattern of chaos or if you've had difficulty controlling your mind and remaining stable during times of stress.

EXERCISE: The Stability Restoration Technique

To begin the exercise, find a comfortable position with your back straight. Then close your eyes and breathe deeply through your nose for two to three minutes. Continue by performing the Orgasmic Bliss Mudra (see figure 9: The Orgasmic Bliss Mudra, page 70). Hold the mudra for five minutes. After five minutes, continue to hold the mudra while you assert, *"It's my intent to center myself in the field of the knower."* Once you're centered, continue by asserting, *"It's my intent to fill my field of the knower with bliss and prana."* Enjoy the process for five minutes. Then assert, *"It's my intent to center myself in my field of knowledge."* Once you're centered, assert, *"It's my intent to fill my field of knowledge with bliss and prana."* Enjoy the process for ten minutes more. Then count from one to five. When you reach the number five, open your eyes and bring yourself out of the meditation.

If you fill both the field of the knower and the field of knowledge with prana and bliss every day for a month, chaos will diminish, and you will feel more stable and secure in your subtle field.

Jose benefited from the technique almost immediately. Within two weeks, he experienced a dramatic change in his attitude, and he began to feel more stable. Even without his sport, Jose reported that he felt calm and in control of his thinking processes. After performing the exercise for an additional two weeks, he taught the technique to Monica and they practiced it together for several more weeks. During that time, Monica confessed that she was having an affair with another man. How they solved this problem and reconciled will be explained in the following chapters.

PART 4

Going from We to Three or More

The birth of a child is one of life's most joyful experiences. It can bring partners closer together and make family life even more meaningful. But as all parents know, the addition of children changes the family dynamic for both the parents and the extended family. For that reason, it creates a whole new set of challenges for both adults and children.

In the next three chapters, we will look into the family dynamic on both the subtle and physical-material levels—and how you can overcome many of these challenges at their root on the subtle levels of energy and consciousness.

We will begin by focusing our attention on fertility. Those of you seeking to conceive a child will learn to enhance your fertility and create a healthy environment that will support your pre-born's development. Parents will learn how to make space for their newborn on both the physical-material and subtle levels and will learn how they can overcome some of the most frustrating childhood ailments.

The bonds that parents create with their child can have a significant effect on its development and the success of its future relationships. We've developed exercises that will help you enhance healthy energetic bonds with your child before delivery and in its first few months of life. By performing these exercises regularly, you will create an environment that will help your child flourish and be able to share pleasure, love, and joy freely in all their family relationships.

TEN

Making Room for Kids

There are many ways that parents can prepare for the arrival of a child. They can prepare their living space and other family members for the event. They can make time for each other and their pre-born by altering their work schedules. An expectant mother can make adjustments to her diet to ensure that her reproductive organs receive all the nourishment they need to ensure a healthy pregnancy. And both parents can prepare for their new arrival on the subtle levels of energy and consciousness.

Much has been written about reproductive health in the last several decades. However, one problem that is often overlooked is the subtle condition of the men and women who are actively trying to start a family.

In the course of working with couples who've had reproductive problems, we've learned that projections of distorted subtle energy and consciousness can interfere with partners' sexual relationship and a woman's ability to conceive. Karmic baggage, energetic attachments, and projections can interfere with fertility and reproduction—so can compatibility issues.

For a man who must sustain an erection in order to impregnate his partner, the ability to perform during the act of coitus is essential. However, a man's ability to sustain an erection and even his potency can be influenced—often in a negative way—by the condition of his subtle field of energy and consciousness.

Erectile dysfunction and premature ejaculation are problems we've dealt with on a regular basis. And we've learned that in most cases, they are created by attachments, blockages, and the intrusion of external projections.

The reproductive problems that interfered with Patrick and Karen illustrate how attachments to ex-lovers can interfere with a couple's ability to enjoy life and conceive a child. Patrick consulted us in 2009 because of his inability to maintain an erection during penetration. The problem surfaced a few months into his relationship with Karen. It had affected his self-confidence and interfered with the couple's plan to start a family. Patrick and Karen were in their early thirties, so age was not an issue. And Patrick assured us that there was no physical problem because he had recently been examined by his doctor. Patrick went on to explain that he loved Karen and was still exceedingly turned on by her, but when they had sex, feelings would appear that interfered with his ability to maintain an erection. These feelings, he explained, would emerge from his lower abdomen as soon as he entered her. Then they would radiate through the front of his body, making it impossible for him to maintain an erection for any length of time. When we asked Karen how she felt about the issue, she deflected our question by saying that she still felt that she and Patrick belonged together and that she enjoyed it when they were intimate. We dug a little deeper, knowing that there was more to the story. It was only then that Karen confessed that for almost two years, she'd been in contact with an ex-lover. She'd received emails from him and spoken to him on several occasions. According to Karen, her ex-lover, whose name was Richard, still wanted her. She quickly added that she wanted to end the relationship because she felt smothered by him. Patrick told us that he'd met Richard and knew that he resented him. He also told us that he was dismayed to learn that Karen was still in contact with him.

After questioning Karen for a few more minutes, we learned that Richard had participated in a cult and that he often prayed to entities (non-physical beings) to get what he wanted.

After examining both Karen's and Patrick's subtle field, it became clear to us that they both were suffering from Richard's projections. The distorted fields he'd projected had polluted Patrick's second chakra field and lower granti. They'd also disrupted the flow of jing from Patrick's kidneys into his eight exceptional meridians.

Since both the distribution of jing and the condition of his second chakra play a prominent role in a man's sexual performance as well as his ability to give and receive sexual energy, it didn't surprise us that he had a problem maintaining an erection.

To overcome the problem, we recommended that Karen end her relationship with Richard. This would accomplish two important things. It would provide closure for both Karen and Richard, and it would take away Richard's permission to interfere with Karen and Patrick on the subtle levels of energy and consciousness. Karen ended the relationship via email, and, on their subsequent visit, we taught both Patrick and Karen to perform Fertility Cleansing.

Fertility Cleansing

In the twenty-first century, it's common for both men and woman in relationship to carry projections of distorted energy from ex-partners in their subtle fields, especially if the relationship ended badly—or the relationship was transformed into a friendship that maintained unhealthy attachments. These projections are often concentrated in the pelvis, sexual organs, and kidneys.

Naturally, projections that disrupt the functions of these organs on the subtle levels will have a negative impact on the energetic condition of sexual partners and their ability to conceive a child. A man's sperm count and the overall health of his sperm can be affected. Projections can reduce a man's sexual pleasure and block the flow of prana through his genitals and kidneys, making it difficult for him to maintain an erection.

Projections can also have a negative impact on the functions of a woman's sexual organs and her uterus during sex as well as during pregnancy. For women, projections of distorted energy and consciousness can also cause a host of collateral problems on the physical-material level, which include severe cramps, bladder infections, vaginal pain, numbness, menstrual problems, a lack of sexual energy, and orgasmic dysfunction. (Please discuss any worrying symptoms with your doctor to rule out a medical cause.) To overcome the projections of ex-lovers and cleanse the reproductive organs before conception on both the physical-material and subtle levels, partners can perform an exercise we developed and have used successfully for several years.

EXERCISE: Fertility Cleansing

Fertility Cleansing is a ritual cleansing performed on the subtle levels of energy and consciousness by both men and women who want to enhance their sexual pleasure and conceive a healthy child. It can have a profound effect on a woman's ability to conceive and her pre-born's development because partners engaged in intimate sexual activities can inadvertently project distorted energy from ex-lovers into each other's field. This can have unintended consequences because a subtle link between the pre-born and its parents is established very early in the pregnancy. In fact, the pre-born's soul seeks out its intended parents as soon as this link is established. Then, a transfer begins—and elements of the child's soul, including vehicles of energy and consciousness, begin to descend into the developing fetus.

Fertility Cleansing can take several days depending on both partners' sexual history, their general health, and the amount of free time each partner has available. In the first part of the ritual, each partner must choose a time when they won't be disturbed by other people and electronic devices. It's best if partners work independently.

In the first part of the ritual, cleansing partners must review their sexual history in order to make a list of their ex-relationship partners who left a legacy of negative energy and consciousness in their subtle field.

For those of you using this technique, it's essential that your list also includes anyone who violated you sexually. People who've violated you sexually seek power and will always project distorted energy and/or consciousness into your subtle field in order to control you.

Of course, not all ex-partners have disrupted your subtle field. So, when making your list, trust your intuition and let your insight and discernment guide you.

One last thing before we move on. The list you create is a work in progress. You may choose to include additional names at a later time. If you do, you can continue to use the cleansing ritual for additional subjects after you've exhausted your original list.

Once your list is complete, you will use the bliss box to release projections of distorted energy and consciousness that have intruded into your kidneys, pelvis, and sexual organs from your ex-lovers—one ex-lover at a time. Then you will continue the process by filling the organs that have been affected with bliss and blue prana.

Those of you who perform Fertility Cleansing should begin by picking a name from your list. Keep the name in mind; then sit comfortably with your back straight.

When you're ready to continue, close your eyes and breathe deeply through your nose for two to three minutes. Then perform the Orgasmic Bliss Mudra for five minutes (see figure 9: The Orgasmic Bliss Mudra, page 70). Continue to hold the mudra while you assert, *"It's my intent to observe the most distorted field projected by* (ex partner's name here) *that is disrupting my ability to conceive a healthy child."* Once you can observe the distorted field, assert, *"It's my intent to surround the distorted field with a bliss box."* As soon as the box has surrounded the distorted field, assert, *"It's my intent to fill the bliss box I created with bliss and to release the distorted field within it."* Don't do anything after that. The distorted field in the box will be released automatically. Although the process is usually instantaneous, it's best to wait a minute or two to ensure that the field in the bliss box has been released.

When you're ready to continue, assert, *"It's my intent to fill my pelvis, genitals, and kidneys with blue prana and bliss."* Take five minutes to enjoy the effects. Then release the Orgasmic Bliss Mudra and count from one to five. When you reach the number five, bring yourself out of the exercise.

We recommend that you perform Fertility Cleansing once a day until all the names on your list have been exhausted and there are no more distorted fields of energy or consciousness that are strong enough to interfere with your ability to conceive.

After they'd performed Fertility Cleansing for six weeks, Patrick and Karen began to enhance their sexual relationship by experiencing their three fields of jing and by performing the Jing Enhancement Technique (see page 124). The three exercises had the desired effect. After performing the exercises for two more months, Patrick reported that he no longer experienced any form of erectile dysfunction and that his sexual life with Karen had reached a new level of satisfaction. We continued to work with them until Karen became pregnant eighteen months later.

After Hanna and Barry had performed the Jing Enhancement Technique for several months, they explained to us that they were interested in having a second child. Hanna was adamant that she wanted a boy. But we explained that there was no form of deep family healing that could guarantee that their second child would be a boy. We went on to explain that they could continue their process of healing by performing Fertility Cleansing. They enthusiastically agreed to perform this technique together. And to their surprise, Hanna became pregnant three months later. Nine months after that, she gave birth to a healthy girl. However, problems developed almost immediately. After Hanna returned home from the hospital, Patty, their newborn, began to scream for no apparent reason. Doctors were at a loss to explain why no amount of cuddling or reassurance seemed to mollify her.

When we received a frantic call from Hanna, we agreed to look into the problem and to see if we could help. You will learn how Hanna put an end to Patty's screaming in chapter 15.

Restoring the Flow of Prana

Restoring the flow of prana though the uterus is another way a woman can enhance their fertility. Two chakras, in particular, support the energetic health of the uterus: the second chakra and the lower physical chakra. The second chakra regulates the flow of prana through the microcosmic circuit between the upper part of the vagina and the area bordering the bottom of the rib cage. The lower physical chakra regulates the flow of energy through the pelvis, including frequencies of prana directly related to uterine health.

To restore the flow of prana through your uterus, you will activate your second chakra and lower physical chakra. Then you will center yourself in both chakra fields and fill them with prana. You can do this in two ways. You can practice the technique once a day as long as you're trying to conceive—or you can practice the exercise for three days before and after you ovulate. In either case, the technique will be the same.

EXERCISE: Restoring the Flow of Prana

To begin the exercise, find a comfortable position with your back straight. Close your eyes and breathe deeply through your nose for two to three minutes. Then assert, *"It's my intent to go to my personal healing space."* Continue by bringing your awareness to your body, soul, and spirit. Enjoy your healing space for five minutes. Then assert, *"It's my intent to activate my second chakra."* Continue by asserting, *"It's my intent to activate my lower physical chakra."* Take two to three minutes to enjoy the effects. Then assert, *"It's my intent to center myself in my second chakra field."* Continue by asserting, *"It's my intent to center myself in my lower physical chakra field."* Once you're centered in both chakra fields, assert, *"It's my intent to fill my second chakra field and lower physical chakra field with prana and jing."* Enjoy the effects for ten minutes. Then count from one to five. When you reach the number five, open your eyes and bring yourself out of the exercise.

Avoiding Desperation and Alleviating Stress

Desperation is a feeling most people would rather avoid. However, it's not unusual for either parent-to-be, seeking to conceive, to become desperate if they haven't succeeded after one to two years. Although there are exercises that can be helpful, we've developed a simple remedy that will overcome feelings of desperation as soon as they emerge. It's called the *Prana Mudra*. The Prana Mudra will do two things: it will overcome feelings of desperation by enhancing the flow of prana through all thirteen chakras in body space as well as the minor energy centers in the hands and feet. And it will facilitate the transfer of prana from your subtle energy field to your physical-material body.

Because of its ability to enhance the flow of prana through the subtle field and the ease of use, the Prana Mudra can also be used to reduce the stress many parents experience during pregnancy, especially if the pregnancy has complications that must be addressed.

One of our clients, Sandy from Toronto, provides an example of how feelings of desperation can overcome someone who hasn't been able to conceive for some time. Sandy was forty-two and her partner Karl was forty-six. For more than four years, they had tried to conceive a child. They tried everything including homeopathy, hormones, and fertility treatments. They even toyed with the idea of hiring a surrogate mother.

When Sandy finally consulted us, she was desperate to find a solution. Although it took her another year to conceive a healthy child, it was her desperation which we dealt with first—since it had begun to interfere with her work and relationships.

Since desperation can only emerge from fields of energy with individual qualities, her desperation became contagious when she inadvertently began to project at Karl, who eventually began to share the same feelings.

To overcome the feeling of desperation, we taught both Sandy and Karl to perform the Prana Mudra, which they used in two ways. They performed the mudra every day as part of their regimen of energy work. And Sandy, who experienced the feeling more often and more intensely, performed it whenever desperation threatened to overcome her. According to Sandy and Karl, the mudra worked better than they expected because, within days, feelings of desperation stopped interfering with their work and relationships.

We also taught Sandy and Karl to use Fertility Cleansing and the Jing Enhancement Technique to enhance their genital health. They performed both exercises along with the Prana Mudra until the birth of their daughter Lena fourteen months later.

Lena was born naturally at home with the help of a midwife. It was an exciting and deeply satisfying experience for both parents, and for us as well, since the exercises we taught them relieved the anxiety and insecurity that could have interfered with the joy of giving birth. Although Sandy no longer uses the Prana Mudra as part of her regular regimen of energy work, she continues to use it whenever the rigors of child rearing frustrate her, or when a lack of sleep interferes with her daily activities.

EXERCISE: The Prana Mudra

To perform the Prana Mudra, find a comfortable position with your back straight. Then breathe deeply for two to three minutes. Continue by placing the tip of your tongue at the point where the gum meets your upper teeth. Next, bring the tip of your thumbs to the inside of your first joint of your index fingers so that they form two loops. Hold the mudra for ten minutes with your eyes closed while you allow prana to radiate through your subtle energy field and physical-material body (see figure 17: The Prana Mudra).

After ten minutes, count from one to five. Then release the mudra and open your eyes. Repeat as needed.

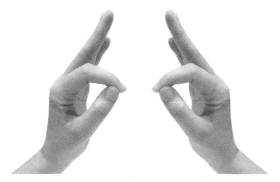

Figure 17: The Prana Mudra

— ELEVEN —
Keeping Your Pre-Born Healthy and Radiant

Even before a child is born, its parents can enhance its health and well-being by reducing the environmental stress a pre-born experiences on the subtle levels. One way to do that is by creating and maintaining a healthy energetic bond with the pre-born while it's growing in the womb. With that in mind, we've created the Pre-Born Bonding Meditation. An expectant mother can perform it on her own, or with her partner. In either case the best time to begin practicing the exercise is at the beginning of the second trimester.

EXERCISE: Pre-Born Bonding Meditation

To begin the exercise, an expectant mother should lie down on her back with her arms at her sides, palms facing upward. Those of you performing the exercise alone should close your eyes next and breathe deeply through your nose for two to three minutes. If your partner is performing the exercise with you, you should both close your eyes and breathe deeply for two to three minutes. Once you're relaxed, assert, *"It's my intent to bring my mental attention to the energy center in my right palm."* As soon as you feel the energy center become active, by glowing or tingling, assert, *"It's my intent to bring my mental attention to the energy center in my left palm."* Take a few moments to enjoy the enhanced flow of prana. Then begin to chant *ohm* from your heart chakra. After chanting for two or three minutes, place your palms on your abdomen with your fingers facing each other.

A partner performing the exercise with an expectant mother should place their palms on the expectant mother's abdomen as well. Hands should not be touching. Continue to chant from your heart chakra while the vibration created by your chanting creates a healthy and enduring energetic connection to your pre-born child.

After ten minutes, stop chanting and bring your hands back to your sides. Continue to enjoy the effects for five more minutes. Then count from one to five. When you reach the number five, open your eyes and bring yourself/selves out of the exercise. Repeat once a day for the duration of your pregnancy.

Chanting Personal Mantras

Chanting personal mantras is another way that parents can bond with their pre-born. We taught this exercise to Sandy and Karl, who practiced it regularly. We also taught it to Hanna and Barry after Hanna became pregnant with her second child.

To begin, pick a mantra that resonates with you (from our list of suggestions) or create a life-affirming mantra for yourself. Then continue by performing the following exercise. Although each parent can perform the mantras on their own—and it will have a positive effect—we've found that it works better when all family members participate in chanting because it will make the birth of a child a family experience, and enhance the relationship that siblings will have with the newborn.

List of Personal Mantras:

1. We are united in unconditional love.

2. You are an affirmation of our love.

3. We are radiant, full of energy and inner strength.

4. You will be born perfectly healthy and full of light.

5. You will know your dharma and share it effortlessly with all of us.

EXERCISE: Chanting Personal Mantras

If you're a pregnant woman performing the exercise on your own, lie down on your back with your arms at your sides—and your palms facing upward. Then close your eyes and breathe deeply through your nose for two to three minutes. Continue by asserting, *"It's my intent to bring my mental attention to my right palm."* Once you feel the energy center become active by glowing and/or tingling, assert, *"It's my intent to bring my mental attention to my left palm."* Take a few moments to enjoy the enhanced flow of prana through your left palm. Then begin to chant the mantra of your choice. After chanting for two to three minutes, place your palms on your abdomen with your fingers loosely apart and facing each other. Continue chanting for ten minutes more while you let the vibration created by your chanting create a healthy and enduring energetic connection to your pre-born child. After ten minutes, bring your hands back to your sides and relax. Then count from one to five. When you reach the number five, open your eyes and bring yourself out of the meditation. Repeat once a day as long as you're pregnant.

EXERCISE: Chanting Mantras with Family Members

This exercise is quite similar, except for the fact that the expectant mother will lie on her back, and the expectant mother along with the other family members participating in the exercise will put their palms on her abdomen. After the energy centers in the palms have become active, the expectant mother along with her family members will chant the agreed-on mantra for ten minutes.

Remain Fearless

To enhance the health and well-being of an expectant mother and her pre-born, we've included some tips in the following text. The first tip is to remain fearless. Excessive fear can be a problem during pregnancy. The Fearless Mudra, which follows, will provide you with a quick and reliable way to overcome both acute and chronic fear. By practicing the mudra when you become fearful, you can quickly calm your mind. By practicing it regularly, you will gradually break down the wall of fear created by fields of distorted energy trapped in your subtle field.

EXERCISE: The Fearless Mudra

To perform the mudra, find a comfortable position, with your back straight. Breathe deeply through your nose for two to three minutes. Then bring your tongue to your top palate and slide it back until the hard palate curls upwards and softens. Once your tongue is in position, bring the soles of your feet together until they're touching. The index fingers are brought together next so that the tips are touching. After the tips of your index fingers are touching, bring the tips of your thumbs and the tips of your middle fingers together.

Keep the tips of your index fingers above the tips of your thumbs and middle fingers. Then bring the tips of your ring fingers together and the tips of the pinkies together (see figure 18: The Fearless Mudra). Practice the mudra for ten minutes. Then release your fingers and bring your tongue and feet back into their normal positions. Repeat as needed.

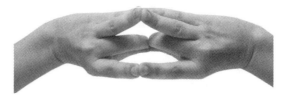

Figure 18: The Fearless Mudra

Increase your Daily Dose of Negative Ions

Negative ions are created in nature as air molecules break apart due to sunlight, moving air, and water. They're odorless, tasteless, and invisible molecules that we inhale in abundance in certain environments. Think mountains, waterfalls, and beaches. Once they reach our bloodstream, negative ions are believed to produce biochemical reactions that increase levels of the mood-enhancing chemical serotonin.

Fortunately, every home has a built-in natural ionizer—the shower. We suggest that you give yourself a negative ion bath by spraying your body with cold water from your shower head at least once a day while you're pregnant.[12]

Think Positive or Don't Think at All

Adepts have a name for the incessant chatter that can muddle your mind. They call it the internal dialogue. We've included a simple technique that will help you quiet the internal dialogue whenever it becomes oppressive. It's called the Beep Meditation.

In the Beep Meditation, every time a thought appears in your mind, you say "beep." Say it out loud; it is more effective that way. And don't struggle with the thought. You don't want to push thoughts away (pushing them away will give them added power). You want the thought to dissipate without it diverting your attention and affecting your emotional state.

EXERCISE: The Beep Meditation

To begin the Beep Meditation, find a comfortable position with your back straight. Then breathe deeply through your nose for two to three minutes. Continue by asserting, *"It's my intent to go to my personal healing space."* Then bring your awareness to your body, soul, and spirit. Enjoy your healing space for five minutes. Then begin to pay attention to the thoughts that fill your mind, and each time a thought appears, say "beep." Stay relaxed when you say beep. Don't say it with any emphasis or force. Remember, you don't want to push thoughts out of your mind. You want the thoughts to dissipate on their own. Continue to beep thoughts out of your mind for about ten minutes or until the internal dialogue subsides. By practicing the Beep Meditation whenever you are distracted by a barrage of thoughts, your mind will become clearer and negative thoughts will have less power to interfere with your well-being.[13]

Feel Good About Yourself

To feel good about yourself, you have to accept yourself as you are Now. To do that, we've provided you with a mudra designed specifically for that purpose. It's called the Self-Acceptance Mudra.

EXERCISE: The Self-Acceptance Mudra

To perform the mudra, find a comfortable position with your back straight. Then bring your tongue to your top palate and slide it back until the hard palate curls upward and softens. Keep the tip of your tongue in contact with your upper palate while you place the soles of your feet together. Next, bring the mounts of Venus (the part of your palm at the base of your thumb) and the edges of your thumbs together. Then slide your right index finger over your left index finger so that the tip of the right finger rests atop the second joint of your left finger. The middle fingers are placed together so that the tips are touching. Once they're touching, place the outsides of the ring fingers together from the first to the second joint. Then bring the inside of the pinkies together from the tips to the first joints (see figure 19: The Self-Acceptance Mudra).

Practice the mudra for ten minutes. Then release your fingers and bring your tongue and feet back to their normal position. By practicing the Self-Acceptance Mudra regularly, you will be able to accept yourself as you are Now. And you will be able to enjoy your pregnancy without judgment and expectations getting in your way.

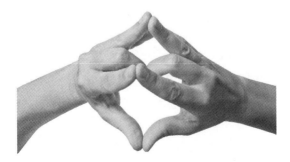

Figure 19: The Self-Acceptance Mudra

— TWELVE —
Overcoming Birth Traumas

All parents hope that their children will be born without complications. However, some parents are faced with unexpected challenges. One challenge that parents can face is birth trauma. Birth traumas always include a physical trauma and a non-physical trauma called a trauma scar. In this chapter, we will look into the energetic events that can traumatize a child and create a trauma scar during and after the birthing process.

What Causes Trauma Scars

A newborn can suffer a birth trauma if the mother has a Caesarean section or a difficult labor, or if the mother's life is in danger during delivery. Of course, not all birth traumas occur during the actual birthing process. A baby can be traumatized directly after birth if it's rejected by its mother or father or other family members—physically and/or psychologically—or if the child is separated from the mother for more than a few moments. Adults can also suffer from trauma scars if they've been physically, sexually, or psychologically abused.

Deloris, a single mother from New Mexico, whose younger child Sebastian suffered a birth trauma during delivery, illustrates how important it is to release trauma scars. Deloris had two boys, Lorenzo and Sebastian. Problems with Sebastian began immediately after birth. He refused to breastfeed and could only be nourished by drinking formula. He screamed continuously, which Deloris found increasingly difficult to tolerate. Deloris became increasingly desperate and feared that she would burn out if something didn't change. As a last resort, she consulted us. We met her at her home and learned that she had had a difficult labor, which had ended with a Caesarean section. She also told us that Sebastian suffered anoxia, oxygen deprivation, during delivery because the umbilical cord became entangled around his neck.

We realized almost immediately that burnout was part of Deloris's problem and that to heal the family dynamic, we had to deal with Sebastian's birth trauma.

Although Sebastian was physically healthy, his subtle field contained several trauma scars that were caused by Deloris's difficult delivery.

To stabilize the situation, we taught Deloris to perform the Prana Mudra so she would have the space she needed in her subtle field to cope with the issues her family faced. Then we taught her to locate and release the trauma scars in Sebastian's subtle field. She quickly mastered the technique and released six trauma scars—four were located in and near Sebastian's throat chakra and the other two by his second chakra. Deloris's work produced the desired result within weeks. Sebastian's screaming subsided and he began to accept his mother's affection more readily.

Unfortunately, the trauma scars in Sebastian's throat had negatively impacted his older half-brother Lorenzo by blocking the normal flow of energy through his governor and conceptual meridians. This was something we encountered in many families we worked with and is consistent with how energetic interactions take place on the subtle levels.

According to Deloris, the collateral effects Lorenzo suffered from his brother's unconscious projections included throat problems, a lack of motivation, and an inability to control his anger, which had begun almost immediately after Sebastian was born. These symptoms revealed that Lorenzo was having problems radiating prana freely from his second and fifth chakras, the same chakras that had been blocked by trauma scars in his brother's subtle field. While Deloris didn't associate Lorenzo's problems with the birth of Sebastian, a subtle relationship always exists between siblings. This means that blockages in one child's field can interfere with their sibling's field, especially if the children live in close proximity to each other. This was the case with Sebastian and Lorenzo, who shared the same bedroom.

When we finally met Lorenzo two weeks later, he barely spoke and was far less animated than a typical boy his age should have been. Sabine attempted to engage him in conversation several times without much success, and I provided him with several toys, which didn't seem to interest him. While Sabine continued to engage him in conversation, I examined the condition of his subtle field. What I found was consistent with Sebastian's condition. Lorenzo had blockages by both his second and fifth chakras. His fifth chakra appeared to have caused him the most discomfort, but experience has taught us that when someone experiences pressure, discomfort, or pain in a traditional chakra, it usually indicated that a more severe problem exists in its companion chakra, which, because of a greater accumulation of distorted energy, has become numb.

The second and fifth chakras are companion chakras, and they share similar functions, including self-expression and access to one's personal space. The second and fifth chakras also regulate person's ability to express joy and to share feelings and emotions freely.

During the session we treated both children by releasing the trauma scars in Sebastian's subtle field. Then we used the prana box to release the blockages that had interfered with the functions of Lorenzo's second and fifth chakras.

In chapter 7, you learned that Irene suffered a significant trauma in childhood when she was sexually abused by her high school swimming coach. She was twelve years old at the time. When we looked into her field, in her first session, we quickly recognized that she carried several trauma scars in her first and second chakra fields.

To rectify the situation, we taught her to locate the trauma scars and to use the prana box to release them. She agreed, but only if we allowed her to do the work in our presence. Like many survivors of sexual abuse, she feared facing the blockages alone and needed the support of people she trusted.

We used the same techniques to treat Sarah, Petra's daughter, whose sleep problem had been caused by a combination of trauma scars that disrupted the functions of her first chakra and cords that had been projected into her field of sleep by her natural father who had abandoned the family a year after Sarah was born.

Trauma Scars

While it's true that most physical symptoms associated with birth traumas are healed with few or no complications, the energetic trauma is rarely addressed. As a result, a newborn may appear perfectly normal after any of the events we described earlier in this chapter—but the trauma will be imprinted in their subtle field as a trauma scar. And it will continue to interfere with the child's development and personal relationships for years afterward.

Fortunately, like Deloris and Petra, you can overcome the energetic effects of a birth trauma by locating and releasing the trauma scars associated with it. In the following two exercises, you will learn to do both. After that, you will learn to restore the flow of prana through the area of your child's subtle field affected by the trauma scar.

Locating and Releasing a Trauma Scar

Before you can release a trauma scar, you must be able to locate it. This won't be difficult because a trauma scar will be located in the same position as the original physical trauma. In addition, a trauma scar will make the area of the physical body where it's located hot, cold, stiff, numb, overly sensitive, and/or prone to physical ailments.

To a person with discernment on the subtle levels, a trauma scar will look like a narrow piece of elastic that has been stretched and frozen in place. It will be clear when it's first viewed because it has been suffused with prana. It's only by looking more deeply into it that you will notice denser, darker energy in parallel bands running through it. These bands are composed of energy with individual qualities. It's these bands that prevent prana from flowing freely through your child's subtle field.

To locate a trauma scar, you will make a journey through your child's subtle field. During your journey, it's important to pay attention to the markers we've already provided as well as your intuition and discernment. It's also important to be aware that a trauma scar is saturated with frozen prana, which means it will block your mental attention. So, if your child has a trauma scar in their throat because their breathing was restricted during delivery, your mental attention will be prevented from moving through their throat and the surrounding area.

Since it will be easier to locate and release a trauma scar when your child is inactive, we recommend that you perform the following two exercises while your child is asleep.

EXERCISE: Locating a Trauma Scar

To locate a trauma scar in your child's subtle field, find a comfortable position with your back straight. Then close your eyes and breathe deeply through your nose for two to three minutes. Continue by asserting, *"It's my intent to go to my personal healing space."* Then bring your awareness to your body, soul, and spirit. Enjoy your healing space for five minutes. Then assert, *"It's my intent to visualize a white screen eight feet* (two and a half meters) *in front of me."* Once the visual screen has materialized, assert, *"It's my intent to visualize an image of* (child's name) *on the screen."* Keep your appropriate senses (sight, hearing, feeling, etc.) open and active because it's by turning your appropriate senses inward, on the subtle planes, that you will perceive the trauma scar more readily.

After you've examined your child's image from eight feet (two and a half meters) away and located one or more trauma scars, assert, *"It's my intent to project myself into my child's subtle field alongside the trauma scar I've chosen to release."* Use all the appropriate senses to move through the area and examine it. Pay special attention to everything you see and feel. Shifts in your emotional state and body awareness can provide you with additional information.

Don't be concerned if you don't find a trauma scar right away. If there is a trauma scar and you remain centered in your subtle field, with practice, its features will begin to emerge clearly.

Once you've observed the trauma scar and you're satisfied with what you've learned, assert, *"It's my intent to return to my original position eight feet* (two and a half meters) *in front of my visual screen."* Release the image of your child and the visual screen. Then count from one to five. When you reach the number five, open your eyes and bring yourself out of the exercise.

After you've successfully located a trauma scar you can refine your ability through repetition. Even if you've had only limited success, with practice, your ability will improve—and, over time, you will be able to see and locate trauma scars in your child's subtle field, your field and the fields of your other family members.

Exercise: Releasing Trauma Scars

In this exercise, you will use the prana box to release a trauma scar you located in your child's subtle field.

To begin, find a comfortable position with your back straight. Close your eyes and breathe deeply through your nose for two to three minutes. Then count backward from five to one and from ten to one. Continue by asserting, *"It's my intent to go to my personal healing space."* Then bring your awareness to your body, soul, and spirit. Enjoy your healing space for five minutes. Then assert, *"It's my intent to create a visual screen eight feet* (two and a half meters) *in front of me."* Once the visual screen has materialized, assert, *"It's my intent to visualize an image of* (child's name) *on the screen."*

Take a few moments to examine the image using the appropriate senses. Then bring your mental attention to the area where the trauma scar is located. When you're ready to continue, assert, *"It's my intent to surround the trauma scar I have in mind with a prana box."* Once you can sense and/or see the box, assert, *"It's my intent to fill the box with prana and release the trauma scar and all the distorted energy fields within it."* Don't do anything after that. Prana will fill the box you've created and release the trauma scar and the distorted energy that supports it automatically.

Once the distorted fields have been released, release the image of your child and the visual screen. Then count from one to five. When you reach the number five, open your eyes and bring yourself out of the exercise.

Continue to use the prana box until all the remaining trauma scars that afflict your child have been released.

EXERCISE: **Zone Method for**
Restoring the Flow of Prana

Once a trauma scar has been released, it's important to enhance the flow of prana through the afflicted area of your child's subtle field and physical-material body. To do that, you will perform an exercise we've developed from reflexology. We call it the Zone Method for Restoring the Flow of Prana.

Reflexology is an alternative medical practice that involves applying pressure to specific zones and reflex areas in the feet and hands. It's based on a system of four zones and reflex areas that serve as an energetic extension of the subtle field. By stimulating these reflex zones in a balanced way, it's possible to enhance the flow of prana through specific parts of your child's subtle energy field and to cleanse their body of residual toxins.

Zone 1: Trauma Scar in the Head and Neck. To stimulate the flow of prana through your child's head and neck, begin by rubbing the top and bottom of the big toe on your child's right foot with your thumb and index finger for thirty seconds. Continue by rubbing the sides of the big toe with your thumb and index fingers for another thirty seconds. Do the same with the other toes. When you've finished the process on the right foot, perform the same process with the left foot. Continue until all ten toes have been stimulated.

Zone 2: Trauma Scar in the Spine and Back from the Waist to the Shoulders. This is the zone where Deloris found trauma scars in Sebastian's subtle field. Like Deloris, you will use the outside of your index finger to rub the inside of your child's feet, one at a time, from the base of the big toe to the heel. This will stimulate the flow of prana through your child's spine and back. We recommend that you begin with the right foot and then move to the left foot, spending about five minutes stimulating the flow of prana through each foot.

Zone 3: Trauma Scar in the Front from the Waist to the Shoulders. To stimulate the flow of prana through your child's chest, midsection, and abdomen, hold your child's right foot with your positive hand (i.e., right hand if you're right-handed, left hand if you're left-handed) so that your thumb is positioned on the sole. Then, using the soft pad on the inside of your thumb, make clockwise circles. Do the same with your child's left foot. Continue working with each foot for two to three minutes.

Zone 4: Trauma Scar in the Pelvis, Legs, and Feet. To stimulate the flow of prana through your child's pelvis, legs, and feet, take their right foot in your feminine hand and their right leg in your positive hand. Using the soft pad of the thumb on your positive hand, rub the heel of your child's foot by first making ten clockwise circles and then ten strokes on each side of the heel from the front of the foot to the back. Repeat the process with your child's left foot.

Sebastian and Sarah benefited from having their trauma scars and blockages released and by having the flow of prana through their subtle fields restored. We recommend that like Deloris and Petra, you stimulate the flow of prana for your child every day for five days after you've released a trauma scar.

PART 5

Helping Your Family Members Flourish

Today's families face a host of challenges that can interfere with the well-being and health of both parents and children. In part five of this book, you will learn to safeguard your family's health and the health of your family relationships by recognizing these challenges and dealing with them effectively on both the physical-material and subtle levels.

One way you can safeguard family relationships is by creating a stable home environment where everyone's needs and personal space are given the respect they deserve. In this way, you and your family members will continue to grow and evolve without the need to restore your psychological and spiritual health later. Another way that you can help your family flourish is to make sure that everyone in your family has an honest and trusting relationship with each other—so that lines of communication remain open and family members remain trusted allies.

You will learn to enhance the stability of your home environment by enhancing trust, honesty, and communication in the next five chapters. And you will learn to enhance the self-confidence and self-esteem of your family members by strengthening your family field so that they have the resources they need to flourish in the modern world.

We also recognize that transitions are part of family life and that there will come a time when your children leave the nest. Although this can be an exciting time for young adults, it can be very stressful for parents. To ease the transition for parents, we've included exercises designed to make letting go easier and to strengthen the bonds of love.

Resentment and regrets can poison relationships and take the grace out of growing old. We've included exercises to overcome these two poisons at their root in your subtle field—so growing old gracefully can be one of the most joyful phases of your life.

— THIRTEEN —

Keeping Your Children Radiant

Childhood is the time when children learn to play, stand, walk, talk, and interact with family members. When your children play with you and other people, they are learning—that they are loved and that they're fun to be around. They are also developing social skills that will enable them to build satisfying, intimate relationships all their lives. For these reasons it's extremely important that they experience a subtle environment at home that is nourishing. One way to do that is to ensure that their wood element remains strong. This will guarantee that your children will remain spontaneous and radiant all their lives.

The wood element is dominant in children from their birth until they reach puberty. According to Chinese adepts, the element wood is associated with various organs of the body, including the liver and gall bladder. Both the liver and gall bladder have a special importance for young children because they support spontaneity and regulate their ability to express themselves freely. In order to ensure that your child's wood element is strong, you can perform the Wood Enhancement Exercise along with them.

EXERCISE: The Wood Enhancement Exercise

To strengthen the wood element for your child, pick a time when the child is lying down comfortably. Then sit nearby, close your eyes— and breathe deeply through your nose for two to three minutes.

Once you're relaxed, bring your hands up to your chest and, with the palms facing each other, bring your mental attention to the minor energy centers in your palms (see figure 8: Minor Energy Centers in the Hands and Feet, page 62). Then bring your tongue to the top of your mouth. Continue by rubbing your palms together until you feel golden prana (chi) ignite in the center of your hands. Experience the flame getting stronger until your hands are filled with its light. Take a few moments to enjoy the effects. Then put your left palm on your child's left eye and your right palm on her/his right eye. Make sure the energy centers in the palms are directly over their eyes. And, if possible, make it enjoyable for your child by making the process a game. Keep your hands on their eyes for two to three minutes. Then remove them and rub your palms together once again—making sure that the flame re-ignites in the center of your palms. When both hands are glowing with chi, place your right palm on your child's gall bladder and your left palm on their liver. Hold your hands in place for another two to three minutes. Then imagine that the golden chi radiating from your palms is filling your child's gall bladder and liver with life-affirming energy. After another two to three minutes, return your tongue and hands to their normal position. After that, count from one to five. When you reach the number five, open your eyes and bring yourself and your child out of the exercise.

Another exercise that will help you to keep your child radiant is based on the resonance of the human voice and the seven traditional chakras. It's called chanting from the chakras. Once you've strengthened your child's wood element, you can use it to strengthen the energetic bond you have with them so that you can effortlessly share what you feel with each other. Begin to perform this exercise once your child is two and a half years old, and continue to perform it as long as they remain interested.

Exercise: Chanting from the Chakras

To chant from the chakras, sit facing your child and gaze at them while you freely share your feeling of enjoyment. When you're ready to continue, bring your mental attention to your first chakra and chant *ohm* in the tone of G. G will create a sympathetic vibration in your first chakra the same way a sympathetic vibration is created in a violin string when a tuning fork with the same tone is struck next to it.

Chant the tone from your first chakra by yourself first. Then encourage your child to chant the same tone with you two more times. After chanting the tone three times, raise the tone to A—and chant three times from your second chakra along with your child. Continue in the same way chanting B for the third chakra, C for the fourth chakra, D for the fifth chakra, E for the sixth chakra, and F for the seventh chakra. The tone for the seventh chakra may sound flat, but it's these tones that will enhance the functions of the seven traditional chakras.

If you're not sure which tone to chant, begin the exercise by chanting the lowest tone you can vocalize—and then shift the tone until you feel that a sympathetic resonance has emerged from your first chakra. The sympathetic resonance, which will emerge as a vibration or glowing sensation at the first chakra gate, will indicate that you are chanting the appropriate tone. You can use the same technique to make sure you are chanting the appropriate tone for all seven traditional chakras.

After you and your child have chanted from the seven traditional chakras, continue chanting from your heart chakras for another five minutes. Perform this exercise once or twice a week for as long as your child continues to enjoy it.[14]

Enhancing Your Child's Chi

With the influence of digital technology and the movement of so many families to urban centers, even young children can become estranged from natural sources of chi, including old growth forests, waterfalls, and large bodies of water. We've been told about the problems this creates from one set of parents after another; even some of the children we've worked with have complained that they rarely go to the beach or walk in the forest. One way to compensate for the lack of chi in your child's physical-material environment is to enhance the flow of chi through your child's subtle energy system. You can do that by performing the Dantian Vitality Technique with your child.

EXERCISE: **Dantian Vitality Technique with Your Child**

To begin the exercise, have your child lie on their back. Then sit beside them in a comfortable position with your back straight. Close your eyes and breathe deeply through your nose for two to three minutes. Continue by asserting, *"It's my intent to go to my personal healing space."* Then bring your awareness to your body, soul, and spirit. Enjoy your healing space for five minutes. Then assert, *"It's my intent to center myself in my lower dantian."* Once you're centered, assert, *"It's my intent to fill my lower dantian with chi."* Enjoy the process for two to three minutes; then assert, *"It's my intent to activate the minor energy centers in my palms."* Once your palms get warm and begin to tingle, place them on your child's abdomen. Hold them there while you assert, *"It's my intent that chi from my lower dantian radiates through my palms into* (child's name)'s *lower dantian."* After two to three minutes, remove your hands and bring them to your sides. Then assert, *"It's my intent to center myself in my middle dantian."* Once you're centered, assert, *"It's my intent to fill my middle dantian with chi."* After two to three minutes, place your palms on your child's breastbone. Hold them there while you assert, *"It's my intent that chi from my middle dantian radiates through my palms into* (child's name)'s *middle dantian."* Continue for two to three minutes. Then remove your hands and bring them to your sides once again. Relax for another minute or two. Then assert, *"It's my intent to center myself in my upper dantian."* Continue by asserting, *"It's my intent to fill my upper dantian with chi."* After two to three minutes, place your palms on your child's forehead. Hold them there while you assert, *"It's my intent that chi from my upper dantian radiates through my palms into* (child's name)'s *upper dantian."* Continue for two to three minutes. Then remove your hands and count from one to five. When you reach the number five, open your eyes and bring yourself out of the exercise.

We recommend that you perform the Dantian Vitality Technique regularly until your child has all the chi that they need to participate fully in their normal daily activities.

Strengthening Your Children's Character

We've seen time and again how a strong, life-affirming character can help children cope with even the most difficult challenges they encounter.

Of course, it's not only children who will benefit by having a strong and life-affirming character. We were surprised when Henry, the successful businessman from Seattle, contacted us again almost a year after his final session with us. He was still in relationship, but had decided it was time to look at his other character flaws, which included a lack of patience and a vindictive nature that often compelled him to get even with people that he believed wronged him. We taught him to practice the Long-Suffering and Non-Harming Meditations, which he performed for several months.

We were invited to his wedding a short time later and learned from Natalie, his bride, that the meditations had worked wonders. We continued to work with Natalie for several more months afterward because of the difficulty she had letting go of her twenty-year-old daughter Elaine, who yearned to study art in Paris. In chapter 18, you will learn how Natalie finally let go of her self-limiting attachments to Elaine and healed the family dynamic.

We've broken good character down into six essential qualities: discipline, courage, perseverance, patience, long-suffering, and non-harming.

Discipline is the ability to stay centered in your authentic mind, your true vehicle of self-awareness, no matter how stressful your internal and/or external environment has become. Family members who have self-discipline radiate prana freely and have the discernment they need to create successful lives and relationships.

Courage is the willingness to defend your personal space on all levels of body, soul, and spirit, even when there is internal opposition from blockages and self-limiting core values—or external opposition from family members, friends, or the institutions of society.

Perseverance will emerge without restrictions of any sort once a person is committed to sharing pleasure, love, intimacy, and joy, no matter how stressful their internal and/or external environment has become. A family member that enhances their perseverance will be able to maintain a positive attitude and a strong and life-affirming identity in the most challenging situations. On the other hand, a family member who is unable to persevere when the going gets tough will become stiff, self-conscious, and sullen because of the distorted energy that dominates her/his energy field.

Patience is the ability to stay centered in your authentic mind and subtle field even when projections of distorted energy interfere with your ability to express yourself and interact with other people.

Long-suffering is the ability to move forward or persevere in activities that are appropriate, even when you must pay a price in personal well-being and/or worldly success. In order to develop long-suffering, a family member must be able to remain detached from the source of suffering long enough to overcome whatever obstacles confront them. That degree of detachment can only emerge once they've learned to discern the difference between subtle fields with individual qualities and subtle fields with universal qualities.

Non-harming is the ability to let go of blame and the will, desire, and/or intent to harm another person in thought or deed. Non-harming means more than "Do unto others as you would have them do unto you." It means saying No to the impulse to get even with people who've harmed you or the people you love.

It's important to note that although the elements of good character appear to be separate, the truth is that they are all connected because they all emerge from the same source, Universal Consciousness. That means you and your family members already have good character. All they have to do is enhance the conditions necessary for their good character to emerge and bear fruit. So, instead of worrying about your character defects and the character defects of your family members, you and your loved ones can practice the exercises we've provided. If you do that, it won't take long for you and your family members to display the benefits of good character—which include a life-affirming identity and a healthier relationship to yourselves, your friends, and your loved ones.

Exercise: Enhanced Discipline Meditation

Problems with discipline are directly related to polarity problems. Although most people believe the universe is dualistic, a universe with only two poles is far too simple to explain all human interactions and all observable phenomena in the non-physical universe. In fact, as you become more conscious of the non-physical interactions, it will become necessary for you to expand your view of polarity to include seven polar fields through which universal consciousness and subtle energy participate in the phenomenal universe. When it comes to discipline, it's the third polar field, the neutral field, that is most important. In the exercise that follows, you and your child will center yourselves in your third polar fields. Then you will fill those fields with prana, jing, and bliss. This will allow you to remain focused and disciplined in a chaotic and ever-changing world. We recommend that you practice the exercise with your child for at least two weeks. After that, your child can perform the exercise on their own.

To begin the exercise, close your eyes and breathe deeply through your nose for two to three minutes. Then count backward from five to one and from ten to one. Continue by performing the Orgasmic Bliss Mudra (see figure 9: The Orgasmic Bliss Mudra, page 70). Perform the mudra for five minutes. Then continue to hold it while you assert, *"It's my intent to center myself in my third polar field."* Next, assert, *"It's my intent to turn my appropriate organs of perception inward on the level of my third polar field."* Continue by asserting, *"It's my intent to fill my third polar field with prana, jing, and bliss."* Take fifteen minutes to enjoy the shift. Then count from one to five. When you reach the number five, open your eyes and bring yourself out of the meditation. Continue to practice the exercise regularly with your child until they have reaped the rewards of enhanced discipline.

EXERCISE: Enhanced Courage Meditation

Courage is a quality associated with the kidneys. In the Enhanced Courage Meditation, you and your child will fill your energy centers in your palms with prana and jing. Then you will place your right palms on your right kidneys and your left palms on your left kidneys. We recommend that you practice the exercise with your child for at least two weeks. After that, your child can perform the exercise on their own.

To begin, find a comfortable position with your back straight. Breathe deeply through your nose for two to three minutes. Then count backward from five to one and from ten to one. Continue by asserting, *"It's my intent to go to my personal healing space."* Then bring your awareness to your body, soul, and spirit. Enjoy your healing space for five minutes. Then assert, *"It's my intent to activate my third chakra."* Next, assert, *"It's my intent to center myself in my third chakra field."* Continue by asserting, *"It's my intent to fill my third chakra field with prana and jing."* Take a few moments to enjoy the shift. Then assert, *"It's my intent to activate the minor energy centers in my palms."* As soon as your minor energy centers are active, place your right palm on your right kidney and your left palm on your left kidney. Placing your hands on your kidneys will enhance the flow of prana and jing through them. That in turn will enhance the feelings associated with courage.

Keep your palms on your kidneys, and have your child do the same for ten minutes. Then remove your hands and count from one to five. When you reach the number five, open your eyes and bring yourself and your child out of the meditation. Continue to perform the meditation with your child regularly until they manifest the courage they need to participate in the normal activities of life without fear or timidity getting in the way.

Exercise: Enhanced Perseverance Meditation

Your child can't persevere when there is a lack of pressure in their subtle energy field and prana and jing can barely flow through it.

The simplest way to increase the pressure in your child's subtle energy field is to have them activate their first and seventh chakras and increase the flow of prana and jing through their governor meridian. We recommend that you practice the exercise with your child for at least two weeks. After that, your child can perform the exercise on their own.

To begin, find a comfortable position with your back straight. Then close your eyes and breathe deeply through your nose for two to three minutes. Count backward from five to one and from ten to one. Continue by asserting, *"It's my intent to go to my personal healing space."* Then bring your awareness to your body, soul, and spirit. Enjoy your healing space for five minutes. Then assert, *"It's my intent to activate my first chakra."* Next, assert, *"It's my intent to fill my first chakra field with prana and jing."* Take five minutes to enjoy the process. Then assert, *"It's my intent to activate my seventh chakra."* Continue by asserting, *"It's my intent to fill my seventh chakra field with prana and jing."* To complete the exercise, assert, *"It's my intent to increase the flow of prana and jing through my governor meridian."* Enjoy the process for ten more minutes. Then count from one to five. When you reach the number five, open your eyes and bring yourself out of the meditation. Continue to perform the meditation with your child regularly until there is a noticeable increase in their perseverance. After that, your child can perform the exercise on their own for as long as they feel it's necessary.

EXERCISE: The Patience Mudra

To enhance your child's patience, you can teach them the Patience Mudra. We recommend that you practice the mudra with them for at least two weeks. After that, your child can perform the mudra on their own until patience has become a normal part of their character.

To begin the exercise, sit in a comfortable position with your back straight. Then bring the tip of your tongue to the point where your gum and upper teeth meet. Put the soles of your feet together next. Then cup your hands together tightly while you press your left thumbs against the outside of your right pinkies and your right thumbs against the outside of your right index fingers (see figure 20: The Patience Mudra, page 186). Hold the mudra for ten minutes with your eyes closed. After ten minutes, release the mudra and enjoy the effects along with your child for another five minutes. Then count from one to five. When you reach the number five, open your eyes and bring yourself out of the exercise.

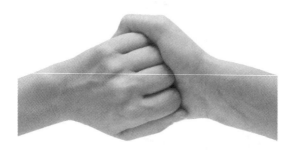

Figure 20: The Patience Mudra

EXERCISE: Long-Suffering Meditation

Long-suffering has nothing to do with suffering. In fact, it's really about the opposite of suffering. It's about the ability to remain steadfast when times are turbulent and/or difficult. In order to remain steadfast, your child must be able to experience joy and manifest it in the world. The second chakra regulates physical joy. The fifth chakra regulates unconditional joy. In the Long-Suffering Meditation, you and your child will activate your second and fifth chakras. After that, you will center yourselves in your second and fifth chakra fields and fill them with prana and jing. As soon as the chakras begin to glow with energy and its essence, you will activate the minor energy centers in your hands and feet. Along with the two minor energy centers in your hands, you have two minor energy centers in your feet, one in each sole. When they're functioning healthfully, they will enhance the flow of prana and jing through the lower part of your body and help you and your child make progress in the world. We recommend that you practice the exercise with your child for at least two weeks. After that, your child can perform the exercise on their own.

To begin the exercise, close your eyes and breathe deeply through your nose for two to three minutes. Count backward from five to one and from ten to one. Then assert, *"It's my intent to go to my personal healing space."* Continue by bringing your awareness to your body, soul, and spirit. Enjoy your healing space for five minutes. Then assert, *"It's my intent to activate my second chakra."* Continue by asserting, *"It's my intent to activate my fifth chakra."* After the two chakras are active, assert, *"It's my intent to center myself in my second chakra field."* Continue by asserting, *"It's my intent to center myself in my fifth chakra field."* Once you're centered, assert, *"It's my intent to fill my second chakra field and fifth chakra field with prana and jing."* Take a few moments to enjoy the shift. Then assert, *"It's my intent to activate the minor energy centers in my hands."* Continue by asserting, *"It's my intent to activate the minor energy centers in my feet."* Stay centered for fifteen minutes. After fifteen minutes, count from one to five. When you reach the number five, open your eyes and bring yourself out of the meditation.

If you practice the exercise regularly with your child you will both remain steadfast and self-confident, even when times are difficult.

Exercise: Non-Harming Meditation

Your child can overcome distorted fields of energy and consciousness that support harmful thoughts, feelings, and actions by developing more empathy for other people. Your children have three fields of empathy within their subtle field; all family members do (see The Three Fields of Empathy, page 97). They're resource fields that supply the chakras with energy. In this exercise, you and your child will fill these three fields with prana and jing and radiate the excess energy and jing through your etheric chakras.

To begin the exercise, close your eyes and breathe deeply through your nose for two to three minutes. Then count backward from five to one and from ten to one. Continue by asserting, *"It's my intent to go to my personal healing space."* Then bring your awareness to your body, soul, and spirit. Enjoy your healing space for five minutes. Then assert, *"It's my intent to activate my upper etheric chakra."* Continue by asserting, *"It's my intent to activate my lower etheric chakra."* Next, assert, *"It's my intent to center myself in my three fields of empathy."*

Once you're centered in your three fields of empathy, assert, *"It's my intent to fill my three fields of empathy with prana and jing."* Continue by asserting, *"It's my intent to radiate prana and jing from my three fields of empathy through my etheric chakras."* Enjoy the effects for fifteen minutes. Then count from one to five. When you reach the number five, open your eyes and bring yourself out of the meditation. Repeat the exercise with your child daily until harmful thoughts and feelings no longer disturb you.

— FOURTEEN —

Strengthening the Family Field

Strengthening and maintaining a strong family field will help to sustain a healthy family dynamic. In this chapter, we will begin by looking at three things you can do to ensure that your family field stays strong. They include keeping your relationship to your family members honest, remaining a trustworthy ally, and maintaining open lines of communication. By enhancing your relationship to your family members in these three ways, you will be able to give them the timely support they need. And your partner and children will know that help is available whenever they need it.

However, most family members know that honesty, trustworthiness, and open lines of communication can be disrupted. That means that many parents find it difficult to provide their children with the support they need when they face challenges outside the home. And many partners with or without children find it difficult to trust one another and share intimacy. Fortunately, all three forms of support have their foundation in the subtle field. That means all three can be enhanced if necessary. To enhance honesty, trust, and communication, we've provided you with a series of exercises that has helped many of the families we've worked with.

You may remember that Jose and Monica consulted us in 2012. Jose had been a surfer for most of his life. But when arthritis prevented him from pursuing his sport, he became difficult to live with. It was during this difficult period in their relationship that Monica had an affair with a local businessman who had competed in surfing events with Jose. The affair continued until Monica realized that without ending it, she wouldn't be able to re-establish the trust she needed to heal her relationship to Jose.

She told us about the affair in confidence because she feared that telling Jose might provoke him to leave her. It was only after she'd performed the following exercises regularly that she felt confident that she could tell Jose about what she had done.

We taught the same exercises to Stephen, Rosalie's second husband. His two daughters Violet and Amanda, who were eleven and thirteen respectively, lived with their mother but spent the most weekends and holidays with their grandparents. Violet and Amanda resented Rosalie and blamed Stephen for abandoning them. As it turned out, the root of the problem wasn't the divorce, although this aggravated the situation. The root was Stephen's inability to share his feelings and emotions honestly with his children.

When parents have problems communicating with their children, it's rarely due to a lack of interest or desire. Rather, the problem is caused by a lack of kidney chi (jing) and an inability to express emotions freely even after they've emerged. This was the root of Stephen's problem with his daughters. His kidney chi had been blocked. But unlike Hanna, who didn't have enough kidney chi to support her sexual relationship with her husband and who inadvertently began to draw energy from both her husband's and daughter's energy fields, Stephen accepted his lack of energy. Unfortunately, by doing that, he became rigid and withholding, which made it difficult for him to communicate honestly with Violet and Amanda. During our original examination of his subtle field, we discovered that, in addition to a lack of kidney chi, Stephen's second and fifth chakras had been blocked. And without their support, emotional energy couldn't reach the organs of expressions in his head where they could be expressed freely. These organs include the mouth, eyes, and facial musculature.

In the following pages, we've provided you with the same exercises that provided Monica the strength and trust she needed to tell Jose about her affair and that enabled Stephen to reopen honest lines of communication with Violet and Amanda.

By performing the following exercises regularly, you will enhance your ability to communicate honestly with your family members and become a trusted ally who will be able to give your family members the support they need when they need it most.

Issue—Enhancing Honesty

Like Monica, most people are dishonest at least some of the time to get out of an uncomfortable situation, to avoid a lengthy or embarrassing explanation, or to evade being wrong. However, being honest with your family members will become easy once you've enhanced your empathy for other people and your ability to express your feelings freely. To enhance your empathy, we've provided you with an exercise designed specifically for that purpose. It's called the Enhanced Empathy Meditation.

You have three fields of empathy within your subtle field (see The Three Fields of Empathy, page 97). They're resource fields that supply your chakras with energy. To enhance your empathy for your family members (and everyone else), you will fill these fields with prana and jing and radiate the excess energy and jing through your kwas, midriff, and armpit cavities (see figure 2: Taoist Subtle Anatomy, page 14). By radiating the excess energy and jing though your kwas, midriff, and armpit cavities, expressing your true feelings will become easier and more satisfying.

EXERCISE: The Enhanced Empathy Meditation

To begin the exercise, find a comfortable position with your back straight. Close your eyes next and breathe deeply through your nose for two to three minutes. Then count backward from five to one and from ten to one. Continue by asserting, *"It's my intent to go to my personal healing space."* Then bring your awareness to your body, soul, and spirit. Enjoy your healing space for five minutes. Then assert, *"It's my intent to center myself in my personal field of empathy."* Continue by asserting, *"It's my intent to center myself in my public field of empathy."* Then assert, *"It's my intent to center myself in my universal field of empathy."* Once you're centered in your three fields of empathy, assert, *"It's my intent to fill my three fields of empathy with prana and jing."* Take five minutes to enjoy the process. Then assert, *"It's my intent to radiate the excess prana and jing from my three fields of empathy into my kwas, midriff cavities, and armpit cavities.*" Take ten more minutes to perform the exercise. Then count from one to five. When you reach the number five, open your eyes and bring yourself out of the meditation. Repeat the exercise every day until you no longer have a problem being honest with your family members.

Issue—Enhancing Trust

To become a trustworthy ally, your children must sense that you trust yourself, and your partner must feel that you're not hiding the truth from them. We've learned that when you lack trust and lie about something, you must divide yourself, which means that the whole truth can't resonate through you. This split is something that most people, especially children, can feel. In addition, lying is always accompanied by a projection of distorted energy, which can impact the people you're deceiving. This exacerbates the problem and can have unfortunate consequences, especially for children. To enhance your ability to trust yourself and the people you love, you can perform the Trust Mudra.

After that, you can overcome the fear of disclosing a difficult truth and the isolation it creates by filling your first and third chakra fields with prana and jing. The first chakra regulates security and insulates you from feelings of isolation and abandonment. The third chakra regulates belonging, trust, and comfort. By filling the first and third chakra fields with prana and jing, your sense of security, belonging, and trust in yourself and your family members will grow stronger, which will make communicating honestly with them much easier.

Exercise: The Trust Mudra

To perform the Trust Mudra, find a comfortable position with your back straight. Then bring your tongue to the top of your mouth and slide it back until the hard palate curls upward and softens. Once your tongue is in position, place the soles of your feet together. Then bring your thumbs together so that they're touching from the tips to first joint. Bring your index fingers together so that they're touching from the tips to first joint. Your thumbs will make a triangle; so will your index fingers. Bring the outside of your remaining three fingers together so that the corresponding fingers in both hands are touching each other from the first to second joint (see figure 21: The Trust Mudra). Close your eyes and hold the mudra for ten minutes. Then release your fingers, open your eyes, and bring your tongue and feet back to their normal positions. Perform the exercise regularly until the trust you have in yourself and the people you love has been fully restored.

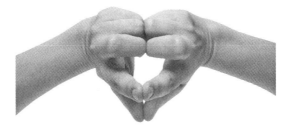

Figure 21: The Trust Mudra

EXERCISE: The First and Third Chakra Meditation

To begin, find a comfortable position with your back straight. Breathe deeply through your nose for two to three minutes. Then count backward from five to one and from ten to one. Continue by asserting, *"It's my intent to go to my personal healing space."* Then bring your awareness to your body, soul, and spirit. Enjoy your healing space for five minutes. Then assert, *"It's my intent to activate my first chakra."* Next, assert, *"It's my intent to center myself in my first chakra field."* Continue by asserting, *"It's my intent to activate my third chakra."* Then assert, *"It's my intent to center myself in my third chakra field."* Take a few moments to experience the shift. Then assert, *"It's my intent to fill my first and third chakra fields with prana and jing."* Take ten more minutes to enjoy the exercise. Then count from one to five. When you reach the number five, open your eyes and bring yourself out of the meditation.

Issue—Enhancing Communication

The ability to communicate is far more complex than simply speaking and listening to the people in your family. Although these are important elements of communication—in a world that includes non-physical dimensions—communicating with your family members includes sharing your feelings and emotions honestly as well as consistently sharing prana and jing with them so that, on a deep level, they get all the love and support they need from you.

The following two exercises, which can overcome the issue, held special importance to Stephen, whose ability to communicate with his daughters on the subtle levels was severely limited. He used them to enhance his ability to communicate honestly and to share more prana and jing with his daughters, who felt that their father didn't care about them. We also taught the same exercises to Alan and Serena. Alan needed to enhance his ability to communicate honestly with Dennis and Kevin as well as his wife Serena.

In the first exercise, you will enhance your kidney jing. In the second exercise, you will enhance the functions of your second and fifth chakras by filling both chakra fields with prana and jing—so that you can express yourself honestly with all your family members.

EXERCISE: The Jing Enhancement Technique

To perform this exercise, see page 124. Enjoy the process for ten minutes. Then count from one to five. When you reach the number five, open your eyes and bring yourself out of the meditation. Continue to perform the exercise every day for three weeks.

EXERCISE: The Second, Fifth, and Thirteenth Chakra Fields Meditation

This exercise will help you communicate more honestly with your family members by enhancing your ability to express authentic joy more freely. The second chakra regulates physical joy, the fifth chakra regulates unconditional joy, and the thirteenth chakra (the sixth chakra above body space) regulates transcendental joy (see figure 3: The Chakras in Body Space, page 28).

To begin the exercise, find a comfortable position with your back straight. Then breathe deeply through your nose for two to three minutes. Continue by asserting, *"It's my intent to go to my personal healing space."* Then bring your awareness to your body, soul, and spirit. Enjoy your healing space for five minutes. Then assert, *"It's my intent to activate my second chakra."* Continue by asserting, *"It's my intent to center myself in my second chakra field."* Take two to three minutes to enjoy the shift. Then assert, *"It's my intent to activate my fifth chakra."* Continue by asserting, *"It's my intent to center myself in my fifth chakra field."* After two to three minutes, assert, *"It's my intent to activate my thirteenth chakra."* Then assert, *"It's my intent to center myself in my thirteenth chakra field."* Once you're centered in your thirteenth chakra field, assert, *"It's my intent to turn my appropriate organs of perception inward on the levels of my second, fifth, and thirteenth chakras."* Take two to three minutes to enjoy the shift. Then assert, *"It's my intent to fill my second, fifth, and thirteenth chakra fields with prana and jing."* Take five minutes to fill your chakras with prana and jing. Then assert, *"It's my intent to radiate authentic emotional energy freely through my second, fifth, and thirteenth chakras."*

Take ten minutes more to enjoy the meditation. Then count from one to five. When you reach the number five, open your eyes and bring yourself out of the meditation. Continue to perform the meditation until you can share your feelings freely with your partner and children.

Stephen performed these two exercises regularly for three weeks. After the third week, he decided it was time to talk with his daughters. They agreed to meet with him in a café, a few days later. After performing the exercises, Stephen had enough space within himself to listen to his daughters with an open heart and to share how he felt with them. They talked for hours and, although Stephen learned that he'd missed out on many of the most satisfying elements of parenting, he couldn't believe how joyful he felt by learning more about his daughters and what they had achieved.

Creating a Circle of Harmony

In 2014, Sandra consulted us. She and her husband Cecil were in their early forties. They had been unable to conceive a healthy child and had chosen to adopt. Their first child, David, was adopted when he was four months old—and, according to both Sandra and Cecil, their experience had been wonderful. David never developed any close friendships and when he was six, Sandra and Cecil decided to adopt a second child, who was a year younger. That's when major problems began to disrupt the family dynamic. Their second child, Harvey, had spent most of his life in an orphanage. He'd been in foster care twice before the adoption—and each time he had been rejected after a short stay. Although the first few weeks were harmonious, it didn't take long for the children to begin fighting and for Harvey to rebel against his adopted parents' authority. The atmosphere continued to darken, and discord soon spread to the parents, who began to argue about who or what was to blame.

During our first session, we realized that the family dynamic had karmic roots that could not be ignored or neglected. Our research into the subtle field relationships indicated that the children had known each other in past lives and had unresolved conflicts that were once again interfering with their relationship.

We felt strongly that the reason the children were brought together again was to resolve their differences so that they could finally enjoy a healthy and productive relationship with each other and their parents. By observing the condition of the children's subtle fields, we recognized that several karmic issues separated them and made it difficult for them to get along. The children didn't share the same soul vibration, and Harvey was jealous of David because he had gotten what Harvey missed most—the affection of loving parents. To overcome the problems, we worked on the children's karmic issues and their influence on the family dynamic.

But first, we taught Sandra, who was on the verge of burnout, to perform the Keep-It-Together Mudra. You will find the Keep-It-Together Mudra in the next chapter.

Sandra practiced the mudra every day, and, in our next session, she assured us that she was no longer stressed out.

Since her condition had improved, we explained that the next step in deep family healing was to create a subtle family environment which nourished both the children and parents. Only then could we begin to heal the specific karmic patterns that interfered with the individual family relationships.

Fortunately, we'd already developed a technique which we'd used in similar situations. We called it the Family Harmony Circle. It was a circle of unconditional love and understanding that family members created to nourish themselves and each other.

We'd already taught the technique to Alan and Serena and their two sons Dennis and Kevin, who continued to perform it regularly. The last time we heard from them, we were told that Alan had stopped judging Dennis and that he supported his son's desire to study art and design in New York City.

The Family Harmony Circle is based on the principle that family members living in the same household create their own unique family field. The field surrounds each family member in the household and fills them with energy and jing. To use the family field to restore family relationships, you must first locate it and center yourself in it. To do that, each family member can perform the following exercise. It's not necessary for family members to perform the exercise together. It's only necessary for them to locate the field for themselves and center themselves within it.

EXERCISE: Locating the Family Field

To locate the family field, find a comfortable position with your back straight. Then close your eyes and breathe deeply through your nose for two to three minutes. Continue by asserting, *"It's my intent to experience my personal family field."* Take two to three minutes to enjoy the process. Then assert, *"It's my intent to center my body, soul, and spirit in my family field."* Take ten more minutes to enjoy your personal family field. Then bring yourself out of the meditation by counting from one to five. When you reach the number five, open your eyes. You will feel wide awake, perfectly relaxed, and better than you did before.

We recommend that all members of the household practice the exercise several times before creating the Family Harmony Circle.

EXERCISE: The Family Harmony Circle

To create and later to enhance the family harmony circle, all family members in your household should sit together in a circle with their eyes closed. One family member can lead the meditation by having all family members breathe deeply through their noses for two to three minutes. The meditation leader should continue by having everyone assert, *"It's my intent to experience my personal family field."* After two to three minutes, everyone should continue by asserting, *"It's my intent to center my body, soul, and spirit in my personal family field."* Everyone should enjoy the experience for another two to three minutes. Then the meditation leader can continue by having everyone assert, *"It's my intent to fill my family field with prana and jing."* Everyone should enjoy the process for five minutes. Then they should assert, *"It's my intent to share the excess prana and jing, in my personal family field, with the members of my family harmony circle."* Everyone should enjoy the experience for ten more minutes. Then the meditation leader should have everyone count from one to five. When everyone has reached the number five, they can open their eyes and bring themselves out of the meditation.

After a more harmonious family field had been created, we taught Harvey to release the distorted fields of energy that he had projected at David. Then David and Harvey harmonized their soul vibrations.

In a follow-up session, Sandra discovered that her two adopted sons had been brothers in an earlier incarnation and that their conflict had been precipitated by their parents, who had sold Harvey to another family as an indentured servant.

To overcome the past life karmic issues, we released the attachment fields the brothers projected at one another when they were separated as well as the distorted fields that supported David's guilt and Harvey's resentment.

FIFTEEN

Overcoming Parental Challenges

In this chapter, we will look into common childhood ailments that can interfere with a healthy family dynamic. After that, we will provide you techniques
designed to heal them. Before we do that, however, we want to provide you
with an exercise called the Keep-It-Together Mudra.

The Keep-It-Together Mudra will fortify you against the frustration, irritation, and annoyance that can accompany chronic childhood ailments. The
exercise will also restrain you from venting your frustration, etc. on other
people—and from dissipating the energy you need to deal with the problem
effectively.

Exercise: The Keep-It-Together Mudra

To perform the mudra, find a comfortable position with your back
straight. Close your eyes and breathe deeply through your nose for
two to three minutes. Then place the tips of your left thumb and index
finger together to form a circle. Do the same with your right hand.
Next, bring your hands together so that the tips of both thumbs and
index fingers are touching. Continue by bringing the tip of your left
middle finger together with the tip of your right middle finger. Do the
same with tips of left and right ring fingers and your left and right
pinkies. Bring the tip of your tongue to the point where your upper

teeth meet the gum next. Then place your feet flat on the floor (see figure 22: The Keep-It-Together Mudra).

Hold the mudra for five minutes with your eyes closed. After five minutes, release the mudra. Then count from one to five. When you reach the number five, open your eyes and bring yourself out of the exercise.

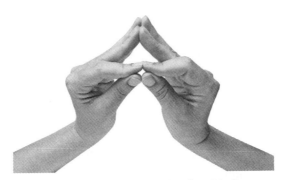

Figure 22: The Keep-It-Together Mudra

You can use this mudra whenever a childhood ailment or a challenging situation elicits feelings of frustration, irritation, and/or annoyance—or when you feel that everything is closing in on you and you need more space, a common experience for weary parents. You can also use it as part of your regular regimen of energy work to enhance your patience and fortitude.

Childhood Sleep Problems

An early childhood sleep problem can create a significant challenge for family members. A lack of sleep can make a child cranky and moody. It can disrupt the child's daily rhythms—and it can disturb other family members, particularly children who must deal with a moody, demanding, and/or depressive sibling. Children who get too little sleep are more likely to have behavioral problems, become depressive, and have difficulties living up to their potential.

One common childhood sleep problem is waking up upset or frightened for no apparent reason. This can happen several times at night or during nap times. Another common problem is the inability to sleep without first eating or drinking something. A child that develops an association with feeding before sleep often wakes up several times demanding food.

Limit-setting problems can also disturb a child's sleep. Limit-setting problems usually begin when the child is about two years old. These problems are closely associated with stalling or the refusal to go to sleep. A child may make one request after another in order to stall the inevitable. Children can become quite creative in order to avoid going to sleep, demanding to be cuddled, to have a drink, or to go to the toilet.

Although authorities have provided parents with common-sense techniques that can help a child sleep peacefully, if these don't work, then the problem probably has its foundation in your child's subtle field.

To overcome sleep problems at their foundation in your child's subtle field, you must release blockages that interfere with your child's sleep cycle. But first you must recognize that human consciousness, which is eternal and is not limited by time and space, extends through various states, in the form of fields, which include both the normal waking field and the sleep field.

Chronic sleep problems are often caused by blockages in the sleep field. These blockages can prevent your child from relaxing enough to enter and remain in the sleep field so that they have a restful night sleep.

In the following pages, we've included two solutions that you can use to solve the problem.

Solution 1: The Calm Kundalini Technique

This technique will overcome all but the most severe sleep problems. It enhances the Kundalini-Shakti, a form of universal feminine energy located by the first chakra. The Calm Kundalini Technique will be most effective for children under the age of three.

EXERCISE: Calm Kundalini Technique

Put your child to bed before you begin the Calm Kundalini Technique. Then sit next to their head and close your eyes. Breathe deeply through your nose for two to three minutes. Then go to your healing space. Once you've brought your awareness to your body, soul, and spirit, open your eyes—but keep them slightly unfocused. Then assert, "*It's my intent to activate my first chakra.*" Continue by asserting, "*It's my intent to center myself in my first chakra field.*" Once you're centered, continue by asserting, "*It's my intent to activate the minor energy centers in my hands.*"

As soon as you feel your hands tingle and/or vibrate, place the palm of your positive hand on your child's medulla and hold it there, with the energy center centered at the hollow between their spine and the back of their head (see figure 23: The Medulla, page 203). If your child begins to move a body part, put your other palm on it while you assert, *"It's my intent that Kundalini-Shakti radiates through my hands and calms (child's name)."* In a short time, the active body part will relax. If another body part becomes active, repeat the process with it. Continue in the same way until there is no more movement and your child is sleeping comfortably.

If your child remains stressed and they keep fidgeting, simply keep your positive hand on their medulla until they fall sleep. Repeat as needed.

Solution 2: The Prana Box

For older children or more resistant sleep problems, you must locate the most distorted field of energy in your child's sleep field. Then you will use the prana box to release it. After that, you will fill their field of sleep with prana.

EXERCISE: Overcoming Resistant Sleep Problems

To begin the exercise, find a comfortable position with your back straight. Close your eyes and breathe deeply through your nose for two to three minutes. Then assert: *"It's my intent to center myself in my field of sleep."* Continue by asserting, *"It's my intent to turn my appropriate organs of perception inward on the level of my field of sleep."* Take two to three minutes to enjoy the shift. Then assert, *"It's my intent to create my visual screen eight feet,* (two and a half meters) *in front of me."* Once the screen appears, assert, *"It's my intent that* (child's name here) *appears on the screen."* Take a moment to observe their condition. Then assert, *"It's my intent to locate the blockage in* (child's name)*'s sleep field that interferes with their sleep the most."* Once you can sense or see the distorted field, which will look darker and feel heavier than the surrounding energy, assert, *"It's my intent to surround the blockage I have in mind with a prana box."* Continue by asserting,

"It's my intent to fill the prana box with prana and to release the dis-torted field within it." Don't do anything after that. The distorted field will be released automatically.

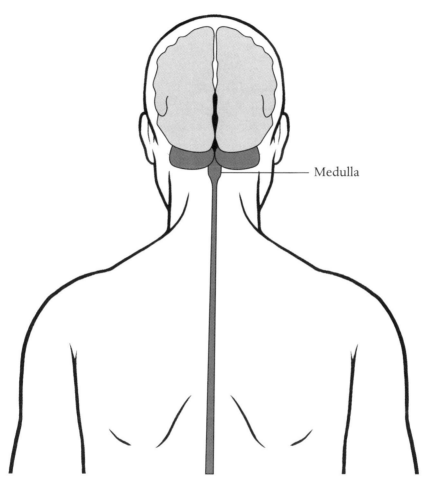

Figure 23: The Medulla

Once you're confident that the blockage has been released, assert, *"It's my intent to fill* (child's name)*'s sleep field with prana."* Take ten minutes to enjoy the process. Then release the image of your child and the visual screen. Count from one to five next. Then open your eyes and bring yourself out of the exercise.

If your child still has problems sleeping after you've performed the exercise, repeat it nightly—always releasing the most distorted blockage in their sleep field. If you continue in this way, in a short time there won't be any blockages left that are strong enough to disrupt your child's ability to sleep serenely.

After we released the trauma scars that had made it difficult for Petra's daughter Sarah to relax, we used the Calm Kundalini Technique to heal Sarah's sleep problem. Petra performed the exercise nightly for two and a half weeks, and to Petra's great relief Sarah began sleeping soundly. She continued to perform the exercise once a week for several weeks longer—and only stopped using it when she was confident that the problem had been solved.

Thumb-Sucking

In many cases, thumb-sucking is caused by a lack of physical and emotional pampering, which in time can disrupt a child's up-down polarity. In most cases, the polarity problem is centered in a child's second and fifth polar fields. A polarity problem in these fields will inhibit the flow of prana through a child's conceptual meridian, the main female meridian running down the front of their subtle field. Although thumb-sucking is the most obvious symptom, the disruption of polarity will also create feelings of insecurity, angst, and—in some cases—abandonment.

Although most people believe the universe is dualistic, a universe with only two poles is far too simple to explain all human interactions and all observable phenomena in the non-physical universe. In fact, as you become more conscious of the non-physical interactions, it will become necessary for you to expand your view of polarity to include seven polar fields through which Universal Consciousness and subtle energy participate in the phenomenal universe. Since thumb-sucking can be caused by the inability to process feminine energy, it's best to enhance the functions of your child's second and fifth polar fields.

The second polar field represents the individual feminine. Fields of energy in the second polar field move inward and/or down through the subtle energy field and physical-material body. These fields tend to be more receptive. They embrace other fields and assert power passively.

The fifth polar field represents the universal feminine. In the fifth polar field, interactions with other fields of energy are a function of vibration, not movement. By enhancing and refining the vibration of the fifth polar field, your appreciation of universal feminine energy will increase, and it will become a fundamental part of your daily experience.

We recommend that you perform the Second and Fifth Polar Field Meditation for yourself to acquaint yourself with these two polar fields before you begin to work on the issue of thumb-sucking.

We developed the following process which includes the Second and Fifth Polar Field Meditation and the Polar Field Empowerment exercise for Gina and Michael because their son Ronald, who was five years old, wouldn't stop sucking his thumb. In our first interview with them, we learned that Michael was a workaholic and that Gina had become the primary caregiver. Without any prompting from us, Gina confessed that Ronald had become the main focus of her life and that she'd probably used him to compensate for Michael's indifference toward his son.

It soon became clear that Gina had inadvertently disrupted the flow of energy through Ronald's conceptual meridian by projecting distorted fields of feminine energy into it. With so much of Gina's energy intruding into his subtle field combined with a lack of physical affection, Ronald couldn't properly regulate his up-down polarity and keep it in balance. That made him overly dependent on his mother. To compensate for the anxiety and insecurity her projections produced, he began sucking his thumb.

Solution: To overcome the problem, we taught Gina to perform the Second and Fifth Polar Field Meditation. This helped her balance her up-down polarity.

At the same time, we released the distorted fields of energy from Gina's fields and dantians that had disrupted her polarity and authentic identity. These included cords and controlling waves. When Gina's polarity had been restored, she began performing the Second and Fifth Polar Field Meditation with Ronald. She worked with him every day for a month—and, by the time he began the school year, he no longer sucked his thumb.

EXERCISE: Second and Fifth Polar Field Meditation

Like Gina, it's best to perform the Second and Fifth Polar Field Meditation for yourself until you're confident that your up-down polarity has been restored

To begin the process, find a comfortable position with your back straight. Then close your eyes and breathe deeply through your nose for two to three minutes. Continue by asserting, *"It's my intent to go to my personal healing space."* Then bring your awareness to your body, soul, and spirit. Enjoy your healing space for five minutes. Then assert, *"It's my intent to center myself in my second polar field."* To enhance your experience, assert, *"It's my intent to turn my appropriate organs of perception inward on the level of my second polar field."* Take five minutes to enjoy the shift. Then continue by asserting, *"It's my intent to center myself in my fifth polar field."* Once you're centered, assert, *"It's my intent to turn my appropriate organs of perception inward on the level of my fifth polar field."* Enjoy the process for another ten minutes. Then count from one to five. When you reach the number five open your eyes and bring yourself out of the meditation.

EXERCISE: Polar Field Empowerment

To begin the exercise sit next to your child. Then find a comfortable position with your back straight. Close your eyes and breathe deeply through your nose for two to three minutes. Then go to your healing space and bring your awareness to your body, soul, and spirit. Observe your child for a few moments; then assert, *"It's my intent to center myself in my second polar field."* Once you're centered, assert, *"It's my intent to center myself in my fifth polar field."* Continue by asserting, *"It's my intent to turn my appropriate organs of perception inward on the levels of my second and fifth polar fields."* Enjoy the shift for a few moments; then assert, *"It's my intent to fill my second and fifth polar fields with prana."* Once the two fields are filled with prana, place your positive hand on your child's abdomen and your feminine hand on their chest. Then assert, *"It's my intent to radiate prana from my second polar field into … (child's name)'s second polar field and from my fifth polar field into their fifth polar field.*" Continue for ten minutes. Then assert, *"It's my intent that the excess prana in…* (child's name)*'s second and fifth polar fields radiates through his/her conceptual meridian.*" Continue for five more minutes. Then count from one to five next. When you reach the number five, open your eyes and bring yourself out of the meditation.

We recommend that you perform the exercise every other day until your child no longer needs to suck on something to feel safe and satisfied.

Gina was so interested in finding the root of her polarity problem that we did a past life regression session with her in our next meeting. The technique we used was simple; we had her go to her personal healing space and bring her awareness to her body, soul, and spirit. Then she used her intent to center herself in the distorted fields that had supported her polarity problem. After that, she performed the Red Thread Technique. She used her intent to create a red thread that connected the distorted energy in her field to the original intrusion of the energy, which took place in a past life. The technique allowed her to travel back through time-space following the red thread to the exact moment in a prior life when she became attached to the pattern.

As soon as she arrived in her past life, she began to observe the activities that had been instrumental in creating the pattern. To enhance the experience, we suggested that she pay close attention to her feelings, the environment, and the people who were present.

If you feel it's appropriate to travel to a past life with your conscious awareness in order to learn how one of your patterns developed, you can perform the same exercise as Gina.

Skin Problems

Skin problems can cause a child extreme discomfort and can have a negative influence on their physical and social development. Research in Germany indicates that, in the last thirty years, the most common form of dermatitis, atopic dermatitis, has increased between 100 percent and 200 percent. And it's now estimated that between 10 percent and 15 percent of all children suffer from it.[15]

Although some skin ailments can be easily diagnosed, others defy a clear medical diagnosis, which means that they probably have a foundation in either the child's colon or in their subtle field.

We've found that it's possible to clear up many skin ailments that defy a clear medical diagnosis by bringing a child's colon bacteria back into healthy balance and by strengthening their metal element.

Solution: To overcome the problem, begin by checking the condition of your child's colon. You can do that by having a blood test performed at a physician's office or a reputable laboratory. This will tell you if allergies are part of the problem. If there are no allergies, the next step will be to analyze the child's stool. This will help you determine if funguses, pesticides, histamines, or a bacterial imbalance have contributed to the problem. If you get a positive result from the analysis, then you must consult an alternative healer or an orthodox physician. If the problem has both a physical and a subtle component or exclusively a subtle component, you can use the energetic tools you've already developed to solve it.

The first step will be to strengthen your child's metal element. To do that, you can fill their respiratory system, skin, and colon with golden chi.

EXERCISE: Strengthening Your Child's Metal Element

To begin, sit close to your child in a comfortable position with your back straight. Close your eyes and breathe deeply through your nose for two to three minutes. Then go to your healing space and bring your awareness to your body, soul, and spirit. Continue by asserting, *"It's my intent to bring my mental attention to my lower dantian, in the center of my abdomen"* (see figure 2: Taoist Subtle Anatomy, page 14). Once your mental attention has been centered in your lower dantian for a few moments, bring your hands up to your chest and, with the palms facing each other, rub the tips of your corresponding fingers together until you feel a golden flame (chi) ignite in the center of your lower dantian. Experience the flame getting stronger until the lower dantian has been filled with its light. Take a few moments to enjoy the effects. Then remove your attention from your lower dantian and assert, *"It's my intent to bring my mental attention to my middle dantian, in the center of my chest."* Rub the tips of your corresponding fingers together again until you feel a golden flame ignite in the center of your middle dantian. Take a few moments to enjoy the effects— which should intensify as more chi becomes available. After you've removed your attention from your middle dantian, assert, *"It's my intent to bring my mental attention to my upper dantian, in the center of my head."* Rub the tips of your corresponding fingers together again until you feel a golden flame ignite in the center of your upper dantian. Take a few moments to enjoy the effects. Then complete the energetic circuit created by your subtle energy system by bringing the tip of your tongue to the back of your upper teeth and by putting the soles of your feet together. Continue by placing your right hand on your child's chest and your left hand on their abdomen. Then assert *"It's my intent to fill* (child's name)*'s respiratory system, skin, and colon with golden chi."* Enjoy the process for fifteen minutes. Then count from one to five. When you reach the number five, open your eyes and bring yourself out of the exercise. We recommend that you perform the exercise every night until your child's metal has been strengthened and the skin problem no longer disturbs them.

Toilet training

Toilet training your child will go smoothly when they feel free enough to hold on and let go at the appropriate times. This may sound counterintuitive, but a child with a blocked energy field—one whose prana does not flow freely—will have difficulty holding on and waiting to go to the toilet. The inability of a child to hold on is usually part of a family dynamic, which includes the inability of family members, including parents and siblings, to radiate prana and jing freely.

EXERCISE: Make Toilet Training Easy

To heal the family dynamic, parents and siblings, including the child who is being toilet trained, must be able to share prana and jing freely with one another. To support this, we recommend that the child being toilet trained, as well as other siblings, step-parents, and/or grandparents, sit in a circle facing each other. Then all family members should begin breathing into their lower dantian. After one to two minutes, everyone should join hands and a designated family member should begin chanting *ohm* from their lower dantian. The other family members should join in as soon as possible. After two more minutes, the designated family member should begin chanting *ohm* from the middle dantian, and all family members should join in. After two minutes more, all family members should repeat the process with their third dantian. Then all family members should assert, *"It's my intent to share my prana and jing freely with all my family members."* Everyone should continue to hold hands for another five minutes while they enjoy sharing prana and jing with one another. Continue to perform the exercise regularly until toilet training is no longer a problem.

Coping with a Screaming Child

For overburdened parents, a child that won't stop screaming can elicit strong feelings of irritation and frustration. A screaming child can create additional problems, especially when other family members and neighbors are disturbed by the noise and the discordant energy. For these reasons, a screaming child can make it difficult for family members to cope. For parents and older siblings who are having difficulty coping, we recommend the Keep-It-Together Mudra on page 200. It will prevent them from becoming overly reactive, angry, impatient, or desperate. And it will enhance their capacity to endure the problem until it's resolved.

EXERCISE: Calming a Screaming Child

Although it can be extremely difficult to soothe a screaming child, we've developed a technique based on reflexology that has successfully treated the problem. We taught the exercise to Hanna and Barry, who were becoming increasingly stressed by Patty's screaming. Hanna performed the exercise daily for two weeks without any apparent success. Nonetheless, we encouraged her to continue because our analysis indicated that the problem had karmic roots. This meant it would probably take time for the shift in Patty's subtle field to be transferred to her nervous system.

Hanna continued to perform the exercise daily, and—a short time later—she began to notice a significant shift in Patty's condition. The screaming became intermittent. And the duration between bouts of screaming became longer and longer. Although Patty remains highly sensitive and will occasionally scream for her mother, eventually the problem became manageable.

To begin the exercise, take your child's right foot in your hands and—with the tips of both thumbs—press and slowly release the solar plexus reflexology point on the sole of their foot until they relax. The solar plexus point is directly below the highest point on the instep (see figure 24: The Solar Plexus Reflexology Point, page 212). Press the reflexology point for nine seconds, in rhythm with your child's breathing. Rest for nine seconds and repeat three times. Then repeat the same process with your child's left foot. Practice the exercise every day for as long as the child enjoys it.

It's important to note that this technique will not produce the desired results if the child is hungry or in physical distress.

Coping with a Child's Will

A strong will is the product of a healthy soul and spirit. It safeguards a child by ensuring that they develop a strong and authentic identity and that they will have the ability to recognize their dharma and follow it. A child's will develops in stages along with their physical body. There are two critical periods during this process: ages two through four (the first period of independence), and puberty (the second period of independence).

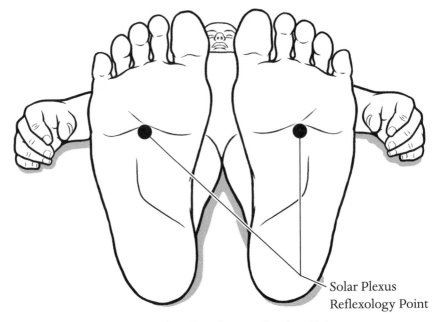

Solar Plexus
Reflexology Point

Figure 24: The Solar Plexus Reflexology Point

Because family dynamics differ, it's possible for a parent, grand-parent, step-parent, or caretaker to block a child's will. An adult who blocks a child's will or engages in a battle of wills with a child often does so because they have a distorted view of parental authority or because they mistakenly take their child's disobedience and/or resistance as a personal affront. Some of these adults have absorbed an authoritarian world-view—and energetic patterns that support it—from their parents. Others retain a legacy of control from past lives.

A sibling can block a child's will as well because of jealousy or because they feel the need to compete with them for attention and affection.

In spite of mitigating factors, a clash of wills between a child and another family member always ends badly for them both—and potentially for other family members, who must find ways to accommodate themselves to it. As a parental strategy, it therefore can't be justified by either family values, societal norms, or the parent's personal experience.

The following family dynamic illustrates how a clash of wills can disrupt the relationship between a child and their mother as well as other family members. Rosie's son Luca was two years old when she consulted us. Rosie was exceedingly controlling—and she took her child's disobedience and/or resistance as a personal affront. She wouldn't let him play without her constant interference or let him go outside when there was a chance that he would get wet or dirty. Although Luca was her first child and she had no formal training, she believed that she was an expert in early childhood development—which meant she rarely took the advice of other parents who had more experience than she did. We recognized during our first meeting with her that she had a problem with her field of will, which had been polluted by projections of distorted energy.

The field of will is located within a larger resource field known as the core field. The core field contains the field of will as well as fifteen other functions of mind including intent, desire, resistance, surrender, acceptance, knowing, choice, commitment, rejection, faith, enjoyment, destruction, creativity, empathy, and love.

If, like Rosie, you're engaged in a battle of wills with one of your children, then it's likely that the flow of prana through the section of the core field known as the field of will has been blocked. If this is the case, you will have difficulty dealing with a child's irrational displays of will, which can include resistance, rejection, disobedience, and anger.

Solution: Although a clash of wills appears to be an intractable problem, the solution we've provided proved remarkably effective for Rosie and Luca as well as the other families we've worked with. It has two parts.

In the first part, you will locate the distorted fields of energy in your field of will that have contributed to the problem. Then you will use the prana box to release them, beginning with the most distorted field. After that, you will fill your field of will with prana. It's important to repeat this process on a regular basis until all the distorted fields that support the pattern have been released and the pattern no longer influences your relationship to your children.

In the second part, you will use the prana box to release the distorted fields of energy you projected into your child's field of will during your clash of wills, beginning with the most distorted field. After that, you will fill your child's field of will with prana. It's important to repeat the process until your child feels confident in expressing her/his will freely.

Rosie performed both sets of exercises for several weeks and slowly let go of her need to control her son and bend him to her will.

Later in the healing process, we taught Rosie to substitute life-affirming core values for the self-limiting core values that supported the pattern and interfered with her relationship to her son Luca.

Exercise Part 1:
Releasing Blockages in Your Field of Will

To begin the first part of the process, find a comfortable position with your back straight. Then close your eyes and breathe deeply through your nose for two to three minutes. Continue by asserting, *"It's my intent to go to my personal healing space."* Then bring your awareness to your body, soul, and spirit. Enjoy your healing space for five minutes. Then assert, *"It's my intent to center myself in my core field in the section that regulates will."* Once you're centered, assert, *"In my field of will, it's my intent to locate the most distorted field that compels me to crush* (child's name)*'s will."*

The distorted field of energy responsible will stand out from the background because it will feel denser and look darker. In some cases, it can also put pressure on you or even cause physical discomfort. Once you've located the most distorted field of energy, assert, *"It's my intent to surround the distorted field I have in mind with a prana box."* Then assert, *"It's my intent to fill the prana box with prana and release the distorted field within it."* Don't do anything after that. Prana will fill the box you've created and release the distorted field of energy automatically.

Some of you may experience a sense of relief and/or a pop. Both indicate that the distorted energy within the box has been released and prana has replaced it.

Once the distorted energy has been released, assert, *"It's my intent to fill my field of will with prana."* Take ten minutes to enjoy the process. Then release the box and count from one to five. When you reach the number five, open your eyes and bring yourself out of the exercise.

Since the patterns may have the support of more than one field of distorted energy, you may have to repeat the process several times. In that case, we recommend that you perform the exercise once a day until all the offending fields have been released.

EXERCISE PART 2:
Restoring Your Child's Field of Will

To begin the second part of the process, find a comfortable position with your back straight. Then close your eyes and breathe deeply through your nose for two to three minutes. Continue by asserting, *"It's my intent to go to my personal healing space."* Then bring your awareness to your body, soul, and spirit. Enjoy your healing space for five minutes. Then assert, *"It's my intent to create a visual screen eight feet* (two and a half meters) *in front of me."* Once the screen appears, assert, *"It's my intent to visualize an image of* (child's name) *on the screen."* Continue by asserting, *"It's my intent to view* (child's name)*'s field of will."* As soon as you become aware of their field of will, assert *"It's my intent to locate the most distorted field of energy that I projected into* (child's name)*'s field of will."*

The distorted field of energy responsible will stand out from the background because it will appear denser and darker than the energy surrounding it.

Once you've located the most disruptive field, assert, *"It's my intent to surround the distorted field I have in mind with a prana box."* Then assert, *"It's my intent to fill the prana box with prana and release the distorted field of energy contained within it."* Don't do anything after that. Prana will fill the box you've created and release the distorted field automatically.

After the distorted energy has been released, assert, *"It's my intent to fill* (child's name)*'s field of will with prana."* Take ten minutes to complete the process. Then release the box, the image of your child, and the visual screen. Count from one to five next. When you reach the number five, open your eyes and bring yourself out of the exercise.

Creating Duality (Good and Bad, Right and Wrong)

When children are born, they live in union with their environment, with their family members, and with Universal Consciousness. It's their experience of union which supports their spontaneous expression of joy and wonder. Creating duality at home, especially when it serves your interests or some social convention, will disrupt your child's sense of wonder and joy by interfering with their relationship to themselves and to everything else in their physical and non-physical environment.

Solution: Duality exists on the physical plane, where hot/cold, up/down, and male/female help us make sense of the world around us. However, duality is much more complex once you factor in the subtle worlds of energy and consciousness. Indeed, for your child to grow up with their spontaneity, wonder, and joy intact, it's essential to avoid creating an overly dualistic environment at home. This means that you should avoid using language that enhances duality. Telling your child that they're good when they do what you want and bad when they don't will enhance duality. Comparing your child to other children will do the same.

To restore your child's sense of spontaneity, wonder, and joy, if they've been disrupted, you can perform the Atman Mudra along with them.

Exercise: The Atman Mudra

To perform the Atman Mudra, place the tip of your tongue on the point where your upper teeth meet the gum. Then put the soles of your feet together. Continue by putting the sides of your thumbs to-gether from the tip to the first joint so that they form a triangle. Place the pads of your index fingers together from the tips to the first joint to form a second triangle. Once you've done that, place the outside of your middle fingers together from the tip to first joint. After your middle fingers are together, place the tips of your ring fingers together. Finally, place the tip of your pinkies together (see figure 25: The At-man Mudra). Take five minutes to perform the mudra with your child. After five minutes, you and your child can release the mudra.

We recommend that you practice the mudra regularly with your child until union and intimacy has replaced duality in all your family relationships.

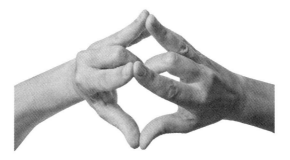

Figure 25: The Atman Mudra

— SIXTEEN —
Overcoming Internal Threats to the Family

Yogic tradition teaches that ancestral poisons can disrupt a person's well-being as well as their family relationships. In the *Laws of Manu*, an ancient Hindu text, we read,

"Individuals are also connected to the larger humanity through space; they are a part of the collectives of nation, race, tribe, religion, and suffer or prosper with the fortunes of those collectives. When a community or a nation sins and faces punishment—war, famine, disease, or an epidemic of drugs and crime—each of its members suffer as a consequence of belonging to that community, even though their personal lives may be blameless. We may call this collective sin, and it also helps to explain people's unequal fortunes. Inherited sin, karma, and collective sin each give a partial explanation for the inequalities of the world within which the individual must find his way. If the punishment does not fall on the offender himself, it falls on his sons; if not on the sons, on his grandsons." [16]

The practice of Yoga is not the only spiritual tradition that makes that claim. In the Bible we read, "The Lord is slow to anger and abounding in steadfast love, forgiving iniquity and transgression, but he will by no means clear the guilty, visiting the iniquity of the fathers on the children, to the third and the fourth generation." [17]

In our research, we've learned that ancestral poisons exist as distorted fields on the subtle planes. These fields of subtle energy and consciousness travel through time and space and can trap children and grandchildren who were not involved in the original karmic activities in self-limiting patterns. Fortunately, poisons of the ancestors exist in a distinct and recognizable form—which means they can be released by an experienced practitioner.

Examples of patterns supported by ancestral poisons include depression, self-sabotage, dependency, greed, abusiveness, envy, jealousy, arrogance, and timidity as well as any self-limiting pattern that you and your children inherited from one of your parents. In order to free yourself and your family members from poisons of the ancestors, it's essential that you locate and release them.

Solution: To overcome poisons of the ancestors for yourself and your loved ones, you must begin by locating the poisonous fields of energy and/or consciousness within the subtle field. Once you or another family member has located a poisonous field, which will look like a bundle of long tubes that intrude into the subtle field from behind, you can use the bliss box to release it. Since ancestral poisons can disrupt family dynamics, it's important to release them from all family members that share the same family lineage as well as any other family members that have been influenced by them.

The importance of releasing poisons was illustrated by the Haldeman family, who lived in Santa Fe, New Mexico. The family's patriarch had immigrated to the United States from Jordan in 1976. Subsequently, he brought his mother, father, and grandmother to the United States. He married an American woman and had three children. All of them lived together in a large two-family house. The poisons of the ancestors could be found in the children as well as their great-grandmother, grandparents, and parents. To heal the family dynamic and restore harmony in the home we taught the children's parents, Abraham and Gloria (it was Gloria who consulted us first) to release them. To facilitate the process, we asked the remaining adult family members if they would participate in the healing process.

There was a long metaphysical tradition in Jordan. And after receiving a positive response, we taught the rest of the household to release the poisons that estranged the grandparents from their children and grandchildren.

Ancestral poisons had also created a gulf between Abraham's parents (and grandmother) and his wife, who practiced a different version of Islam. They eventually agreed to participate in the healing process. And once we were satisfied that enough poisons had been released, we taught everyone in the household as well as Abraham's parents and grandmother to perform the Family Harmony Circle so that they could find common ground with one another.

We didn't hear from the Haldeman family for some time. But in 2016, Abraham contacted us and explained that the family harmony circle had worked wonders. Then he asked us if we would work with his grandmother who had been diagnosed with cancer and was desperate to overcome her resentments before she died. We agreed and met with her several times. In chapter 18, you will learn how she prepared herself for the afterlife by overcoming both her resentments and regrets.

To perform the Family Harmony Circle with your family members, see page 198. We recommend that you perform the exercise after you've released the poisons that were interfering with the well-being of your family.

Exercise:
Releasing Poisons of the Ancestors

To begin this exercise, find a comfortable position with your back straight. Breathe deeply through your nose for two to three minutes. Then choose a self-limiting pattern or blockage that your child shares with one of its natural parents. Keep it in mind. Then count backward from five to one and from ten to one. Use the Orgasmic Bliss Mudra to bring bliss into your conscious awareness (see figure 9: The Orgasmic Bliss Mudra, page 70). Hold the mudra and assert, *"It's my intent to create a visual screen eight feet* (two and a half meters) *in front of me."* Once the screen appears, assert, *"It's my intent to visualize an image of* (child's name) *on the screen in front of me."* Continue by asserting, *"It's my intent to experience* (see and feel) *the poison of the ancestors that is the foundation of the self-limiting issue I have in mind."* The poisonous field will look like a bundle of long tubes that intrude into your child's subtle field. As soon as the poisonous field appears, assert, *"It's my intent to surround the poisonous field I have in mind with a bliss box."* Then assert, *"It's my intent to fill the bliss box with bliss and release all the ancestral poisons in the form of fields within it.*" Don't do anything after that. The poisonous fields will be released automatically.

As soon as the ancestral poison has been released, your child will experience a sense of relief, which is often accompanied by a pop that indicates that the only thing that remains in the bliss box is bliss.

To continue, release the bliss mudra, the image of your child, and the visual screen. Then count from one to five. When you reach the number five, open your eyes and bring yourself out of the exercise. We recommend that you perform the exercise while your child sleeps. Then get feedback from them the next morning.

Since most children have inherited several poisonous fields from their ancestors, you may have to perform the same technique several times in order to release all the ancestral poisons in your child's subtle field. Since most people inherited poisons of the ancestors when they were children, the process will be the same for adults.

Past Life Attachments

Past life attachments create patterns that can affect parents and children and interfere with a healthy family dynamic. That's because they create "blind spots" that disrupt motivation, enthusiasm, and concentration. They can also make it difficult for a person to sleep peacefully and to express their authentic emotions freely. Blind spots that have become large enough can also occupy a significant amount of space on the subtle levels, making it difficult for a person under their influence to empathize with their family members and communicate freely.

The most common past life attachments are cords, attachment fields, and clinging fields. After examining Luca's subtle field, it became clear that Rosie had projected several cords into his field on the dimensions regulated by his second and fourth chakras.

Cords are fields of dense energy with individual qualities that closely resemble long, thin tubes. The tubes are hollow, which means that distorted energy can be projected through them into another person's subtle field. When a family suffers from a past life attachment in the form of a cord, they can remain attached to someone who is not incarnated but who still continues to influence them.

Attachment fields normally have a long, rectangular shape and will be extremely dense and sticky. It's because of these qualities that an attachment field can easily penetrate a person's energy field.

A person's motive for projecting an attachment field will be to compel someone to bond with them in an unhealthy way.

An attachment field acts like a computer virus: it disrupts a person's decision-making process by introducing powerful feelings and desires into his or her energy field. A person who is being influenced by one or more attachment fields will have difficulty remaining centered in their authentic mind. In addition, they will have difficulty feeling and expressing their normal functions of mind, including desire and will.[18]

Clinging fields are projected by people who feel compelled to hold on to another person. Once they've been projected, they will attach themselves to a surface boundary and hold on to it. In some cases, they can connect two people together for lifetimes. They are irregularly shaped but tend to spread out on the surface boundary as soon as they've attached themselves to it. Once they have attached themselves to a surface boundary, they must be released since they won't normally let go on their own. Clinging fields can make it difficult for someone to sense the external world and to form or maintain an authentic identity.

Solution: Family members that suffer from the effects of blind spots created by past life attachments such as cords, attachment fields, and clinging fields can be healed using the techniques of deep family healing. The healing process has two parts. First you must determine if you or a family member suffers from a past life attachment. Then you can use the prana box to release it.

EXERCISE: Releasing Cords

To release a past life attachment created by a cord, you must begin by choosing a negative emotion, feeling, or sensation that consistently influences your well-being but doesn't appear to have a cause-and-effect relationship to what you are doing. Hate, jealousy, and envy are examples of emotions. Disappointment, fear, and resentment are examples of feelings. Pressure, exhaustion, and phantom pain are examples of sensations. These experiences are in fact fields of distorted energy that consistently interfere with your ability to share the universal qualities of prana (chi) with your family members. After you've made your choice, find a comfortable position with your back straight. Then close your eyes and breathe deeply through your nose for two to three minutes. Count backward from five to one and from ten to one. Then assert, *"It's my intent to go to my personal healing space."* Continue by bringing your awareness to your body, soul, and spirit. Enjoy your healing space for five minutes. Then assert, *"It's my intent to become aware of the cord that is responsible for the* (emotion, feeling, or sensation) *I've chosen to release."* Take a moment to observe the cord. It will be long and thin and will extend outward from your energy field. After you've examined the cord, assert, *"It's my intent to surround the cord I have in mind with a prana box."* Then assert, *"It's my intent to fill the prana box with prana and to release the cord and its source and extensions."* As soon as the cord has been released, you will feel a shift in your energetic conditions. Pressure will diminish. And you will be able to share more prana freely with the people you love.

Once you've released the cord, release the prana box and the visual screen. Then take ten minutes to enjoy the effects. After ten minutes, count from one to five. When you reach the number five, open your eyes and bring yourself out of the exercise. Continue to perform the exercise until all the cords that attach you to the past have been released.

EXERCISE: Releasing Attachment Fields

In order to release an attachment field that traps you in the past, you will begin by choosing a desire, need, or obsession that compels you to do things that are self-limiting and antagonistic to healthy family relationships.

After you've made your choice, find a comfortable position with your back straight. Then close your eyes and breathe deeply through your nose for two to three minutes. Count backward from five to one and from ten to one. Then assert, *"It's my intent to go to my personal healing space.*" Continue by bringing your awareness to your body, soul, and spirit. Enjoy your healing space for five minutes. Then assert, "*It's my intent to become aware of the attachment field that I've chosen to release.*" Take a moment to observe the attachment field. It will have a long, rectangular shape. And it will be heavy, sticky, and denser than the energy surrounding it. After you've examined the attachment field, assert, "*It's my intent to surround the attachment field I have in mind with a prana box.*" Then assert, "*It's my intent to fill the prana box with prana and to release the attachment field and its source and extensions.*" Don't do anything after that. The attachment field will be released automatically. As soon as the attachment has been released, you will feel a shift in your energetic condition. Pressure will diminish. Prana will flow more freely and you will experience a renewed sense of freedom.

Once you've released the attachment field, release the prana box and the visual screen. Then take ten minutes to enjoy the effects. After ten minutes, count from one to five. When you reach the number five, open your eyes and bring yourself out of the exercise. Continue to perform the exercise until you've released all the attachment fields that limit your freedom.

EXERCISE: Releasing Clinging Fields

Clinging fields trap you inside yourself without enough space to express your feelings and shift your awareness from one point of your body space to another. In order to release a clinging field that traps you in the past, you must use your discernment to locate it. Clinging fields that connect you to the past will look like thick planks of wood or metal that intrude into the back of your subtle field. They will prevent you from feeling the area where they're located and they will put pressure, create lumps, and cause muscle tension in your physical-material, physical, and/or etheric body.

To release a clinging field that connects you to the past, choose an area of your body that is hard, numb, or which prevents your mental attention from moving through it. Keep it in mind and find a comfortable position with your back straight. Then close your eyes next and breathe deeply through your nose for two to three minutes. Count backward from five to one and from ten to one. Then assert, *"It's my intent to go to my personal healing space."* Continue by bringing your awareness to your body, soul, and spirit. Enjoy your healing space for five minutes. Then assert, *"It's my intent to become aware of the clinging field that I've chosen to release."* Once you can see or sense the clinging field, assert, *"It's my intent to surround the clinging field I have in mind with a prana box."* Then assert, *"It's my intent to fill the prana box with prana and to release the clinging field and its source and extensions."* Don't do anything after that. The clinging field will be released automatically. As soon as the blockage has been released, you will feel a shift in your energetic condition. Pressure will diminish. Prana will flow more freely. And you will experience a renewed sense of freedom.

Once you've released the clinging field, release the prana box and the visual screen. Then take ten minutes to enjoy the effects. After ten minutes, count from one to five. When you reach the number five, open your eyes and bring yourself out of the exercise. Continue to perform the exercise until you've released all the clinging fields that have limited your personal freedom.

Issue: Rejection by Family Members

Children who are different in some way, who don't meet the expectations of family members, or who are members of patchwork families can be rejected by one or more of their family members. This can disrupt self-esteem and create a longing for acceptance. In extreme cases, the child may internalize the feelings of rejection—and neglect their own needs or sabotage themselves in order to get the attention and validation they need. Rejection is not only an issue for children. Adults who were rejected or abandoned as children or who were mobbed and/or rejected as an adult can also suffer from symptoms that interfere with their family relationships.

Solution: Teach your child the Self-Acceptance Mudra and the Self-Esteem Mudra, or perform them yourself if you were rejected, abandoned, or mobbed. Perform the Self-Acceptance Mudra with your child in the morning and the Self-Esteem Mudra at night until you and/or your child overcome the longing for acceptance and the feelings of rejection.

EXERCISE: The Self-Acceptance Mudra

To perform the mudra, go to chapter 11 (see figure 19: The Self-Acceptance Mudra, page 166).

Practice the mudra for ten minutes by yourself or with your child. Then release your fingers and bring your tongue and feet back to their normal position. By practicing the Self-Acceptance Mudra regularly on your own or with your child, you will be able to accept yourself as you are Now. That will bring you one step closer to overcoming the feelings associated with rejection and neglect.

EXERCISE: The Self-Esteem Mudra

Practice the mudra on your own or with your child regularly until your self-esteem has been restored (see figure 16: The Self-Esteem Mudra, page 141).

Issue: Separation and Divorce

Separation and divorce can be traumatic for children of any age. It fosters feelings of abandonment, loss, and guilt that can continue to plague a child for years.

Judith Wallerstein was a psychologist and researcher who created a twenty-five-year study on the effects of divorce on the children involved. Interviewing them after eighteen months and then five, ten, fifteen, and twenty-five years after the divorce, she expected to find that they had bounced back. But what she found was dismaying: even twenty-five years after the divorce, these children continued to experience substantial expectations of failure, fear of loss, fear of change, and fear of conflict.

The children in Wallerstein's study were especially challenged when they began to form their own romantic relationships. As Wallerstein explains, "Contrary to what we have long thought, the major impact of divorce does not occur during childhood or adolescence. Rather, it rises in adulthood as serious romantic relationships move center stage..." As Wallerstein put it, "The kids [in my study] had a hard time remembering the pre-divorce family... but what they remembered about the post-divorce years was their sense that they had indeed been abandoned by both parents and that their nightmare [of abandonment] had come true." [19]

Fortunately, the distorted fields that create feelings or abandonment and self-sabotage can be released. And as we've learned, divorce and estrangement from a loved one can be part of an ongoing karmic relationship that may have its roots in a past life. Therefore, by dealing effectively with the challenge divorce creates on the subtle level, a family member may be resolving a past-life conflict that has plagued them for more than one lifetime.

Solution: In order to overcome the negative feelings that divorce creates as well as to support the healthy expression of grief, which is an essential part of the healing process, we've included two techniques that will help a child or adult substitute longing for the absent parent into yearning for the divine masculine ("purusha") and/or divine feminine ("prakriti").

Our work with Sebrina illustrates how devastating a divorce can be for a grown child. Sebrina lived in Rome and contacted us through our publisher. She'd been married for two years and had become desperate because her husband, Philip—who was a musician—was often away for weeks on tour. Although she knew that he would be away from home regularly before she married him—and she was convinced that he would be true to her—she struggled with feelings of neglect and abandonment. Even when he was at home, she found it difficult to deal with these feelings. Within months of their marriage, she'd begun to nag him in an attempt to change his behavior. This led to fights and a breakdown of intimacy. It was only after she'd been propositioned by another man who'd promised to give her everything she needed that she consulted us.

During our first session, Sebrina told us that she often thought about leaving her husband. When we asked her why she hadn't done it, she replied, "I was six when my parents were divorced, and I can't leave him as long as I believe that my feelings have more to do with that event than anything my husband has done."

The transition between five and seven years of age is critical for children. It's the time when they reach out to the parent of the opposite sex for nourishment and look to them as a role model for their subsequent relationships.

When she began to work with us, Sebrina put her relationship decisions on hold. Then she contacted her biological father, whom she hadn't spoken to in eight years, and told him how the divorce had affected her. Telling him the truth after so many years enhanced her determination to resolve the issue and save her marriage.

We examined the condition of her subtle field next—looking specifically at the attachments which continued to connect her to her father. We discovered several cords and attachment fields that her father had projected at her as well as several cords she had projected at him as a child. We taught her to release the cords and attachment fields her father had projected into her field first. She spent several weeks working through them. Then we had her release the cords she projected at him. These cords were concentrated in her first, third, and fifth chakra fields, precisely the fields that regulate security, trust, contentment, belonging, and joy.

Once the cords were released, we taught Sebrina to perform the Purusha Field Meditation, which she began to practice along with her husband. They practiced it together for two weeks, and she continued on her own for six more weeks. In her last meeting with us, she explained that the feelings of neglect and abandonment no longer disturbed her and that she and her husband had decided to start a family.

Although Sebrina was an adult when she began to work with us, the same feelings can afflict any child whose parents have separated or divorced. In the following text, we've included the Purusha Field Meditation as well as the Prakriti Field Meditation. The appropriate exercise will help both children and adults overcome the negative effects of separation and divorce.

Perform the Prakriti Field Meditation for two weeks with your child if the estranged parent is the child's mother. Perform the Purusha Field Meditation with your child for two weeks if the estranged parent is the child's father. After the first two weeks, your child can continue to perform the appropriate exercise on their own until longing for the estranged parent has been transformed into the yearning for the universal masculine or feminine.

EXERCISE: The Prakriti Field Meditation

To begin the Prakriti Field Meditation, find a comfortable position with your back straight. Close your eyes and breathe deeply through your nose for two to three minutes. Then count backward from five to one and from ten to one. Continue by asserting, *"It's my intent to go to my personal healing space."* Then bring your awareness to your body, soul, and spirit. Enjoy your healing space for five minutes. Then assert, *"It's my intent to center myself in my prakriti field."* Continue by asserting, *"It's my intent to turn my organs of perception inward in my prakriti field."* After a few moments, your orientation will shift, and you'll become aware of a large cavity that interpenetrates your physical-material body. This cavity is the prakriti field. From your new vantage point—within the field of prakriti—you will become aware of the creative power of universal feminine energy. Continue by asserting, *"It's my intent to fill my prakriti field with prana and jing."* Take fifteen minutes to enjoy the experience. Then count from one to five. When you reach the number five, open your eyes and bring yourself out of the meditation. Repeat the exercise every day with your child until the longing for the estranged parent has been transformed into yearning for the divine feminine.

The more often your child practices the Prakriti Field Meditation, the greater the benefits will be—and the easier it will be for your child to overcome the negative effects of divorce.[20]

EXERCISE: The Purusha Field Meditation

To begin the Purusha Field Meditation, find a comfortable position with your back straight. Close your eyes and breathe deeply through your nose for two to three minutes. Then count backward from five to one and from ten to one. Perform the Orgasmic Bliss Mudra to bring bliss into your conscious awareness (see figure 9: The Orgasmic Bliss Mudra, page 70). Hold the mudra while you assert, *"It's my intent to center myself in my purusha field."* Continue by asserting, *"It's my intent to turn my organs of perception inward in my purusha field."* After a few moments, your orientation will shift, and you'll become aware of a large cavity that interpenetrates your physical-material body. This cavity is the purusha field. From your new vantage point—within the purusha field—you will become aware of the profound sense of union and peace that are hallmarks of the field. Continue by asserting, *"It's my intent to fill my purusha field with bliss."* Take fifteen minutes to enjoy the experience. Then release the Orgasmic Bliss Mudra and count from one to five. When you reach the number five, open your eyes and bring yourself out of the meditation. Repeat the exercise every day with your child until longing for the estranged parent has been transformed into yearning for the divine masculine.

The more often you practice the Purusha Field Meditation, the greater the benefits will be—and the easier it will be for your child to overcome the negative effects of divorce.

— SEVENTEEN —
Overcoming External Threats to the Family

One of the fundamental principles of metaphysics and deep family healing states is, "as above so below; as below so above." This means that internal threats as well as external threats can disrupt your family dynamic. Fortunately, parents and children can defend themselves from outside threats that disrupt their family dynamic by enhancing the flow of jing through their field.

From the Taoists, we've learned that you and your family members can protect yourself from intrusions of "evil chi" by enhancing the flow of jing through your exceptional meridians. Evil chi is the same as energy with individual qualities, which can be projected from one person to another. When evil chi is projected with enough force by someone who has strong feelings about you, it can get stuck inside your subtle field. Then it can disrupt your family relationships by interfering with the flow of chi and jing through the organs of your subtle field.

To prevent this from happening, you and your family members must empower yourselves by strengthening your exceptional meridians (see figure 14: The Eight Exceptional Meridians, page 127–130). You can do that by performing a technique that will enhance the amount of jing in your exceptional meridians. It's called the Boundary Safety Net—and it is effective for family members of all ages. By creating the Boundary Safety Net for your family, you will create a barrier that will protect everyone in your household from evil chi, the intrusion of distorted fields, and the negative influence of non-physical beings.

We taught this exercise to Rosalie and Stephen, who were being disturbed by Stephen's ex-wife Miriam and her parents as well as Stephen's two adolescent daughters, Violet and Amanda, who were eleven and thirteen respectively. Violet and Amanda lived with their mother, but spent most weekends and holidays with their grandparents Sam and Bettina, who also resented Rosalie, and whose resentment and general hostility continually influenced the family dynamic. As you already learned, Violet and Amanda had reconciled with their father. Nonetheless, they still blamed Rosalie for stealing their father away.

Solving the problem proved difficult because of the shifting subtle environment. Nonetheless, by using the exercises that you will learn to perform in the following text, Rosalie and Stephen were able to protect themselves from the intrusions that had been interfering with their relationship to one another and to their daughter Sarah.

The intrusions interfered primarily with Rosalie and Stephen's sexual relationship and with their ability to experience intimacy with each other and with Sarah. They also influenced Rosalie and Stephen's inability to express authentic emotions because the intrusions had polluted the couple's personal space on the non-physical levels.

We also taught the exercise to Hanna and Barry, who had restored the flow of jing through their subtle fields but were still being projected at by Hanna's ex-colleague. Since they both suffered from the projections, they performed the exercise together. Within a few days, they were receiving the full benefits of the exercise. Projections ceased to disturb them, and their inner strength, which had been diminished by the projections, was almost entirely restored.

EXERCISE: The Boundary Safety Net

You can perform this exercise on your own, although we recommend that you perform it as a group with all the family members in your household.

To begin the exercise, find a comfortable position with your back straight. Close your eyes and breathe deeply through your nose for two to three minutes. Then count backward from five to one and from ten to one. Continue by asserting, *"It's my intent to go to my personal healing space."* Then bring your awareness to your body, soul, and spirit. Enjoy your healing space for five minutes. Then assert, *"It's my intent to center myself in my three fields of jing* (eternal, external, and internal)." Once you're centered, continue by asserting, *"It's my intent to fill my three fields of jing with jing."* Take five minutes to enjoy the process. Then continue by asserting, *"It's my intent that jing from my three fields of jing fill my kidneys."* Take another five minutes to experience the transfer of jing. Then assert, *"It's my intent that jing from my kidneys fills my eight exceptional meridians and creates a boundary safety net around my subtle field."* Take ten minutes to feel jing radiate through your exceptional meridians and from there throughout your subtle field.

After ten minutes, count from one to five. When you reach the number five, open your eyes and bring yourself out of the meditation. Repeat the exercise every day until you and your family members are no longer disturbed by external intrusions.

Issue: The Media and Social Networking

Your child's authentic mind is composed of three essential elements. On the physical level, it includes the brain and nervous system as well as the chemicals in the body, including hormones that influence its development.

On the non-physical level, the mind includes the subtle field of energy and consciousness, its organs and vehicles—and the prana (chi), jing, and consciousness that nourish them. The combination of physical and non-physical elements creates the third part of the human mind—the network. All three parts have their own unique capabilities and needs.

The network is particularly important to children because it includes the connections the mind has to its individual parts and to things beyond itself. This includes consciousness and energy—as well as attachments to other people, non-physical beings, and their projections.

Texting, chatting, computer games, and hours spent with social media disrupt the normal chemistry of the brain (particularly a child's developing brain). In addition, they can disrupt the ability of the brain and subtle field to integrate their activities and to make healthy connections.

Researchers have described time spent with social media, texting, multitasking, etc. as a form of violence against the mind because after a person has immersed themselves for a short time, their brain begins to resemble the brain of a person with an addictive personality. This can be devastating for a child since the brain affects the network—and the network's primary activity is to communicate with people in a holistic way.[21]

Solution: While banning the use of social media and smart phones at certain times, such as during meals, may enhance family relationships, it won't solve the underlying problem, which is the disruption of the network. The best way to do that is to heal the functions of mind that are being disrupted or blocked by the excessive use of digital media. The Core Field Meditation is designed to do that.

We recommend that you perform the Core Field Meditation with your family members until their functions of mind have been restored to radiant good health.

EXERCISE: Core Field Meditation

To begin the exercise, close your eyes and breathe deeply through your nose for two to three minutes. Then count backward from five to one and from ten to one. Perform the Orgasmic Bliss Mudra to bring bliss into your conscious awareness (see figure 9: The Orgasmic Bliss Mudra, page 70). Hold the mudra while you assert, *"It's my intent to go to my personal healing space."* Then bring your awareness to your body, soul, and spirit. Enjoy your healing space for five minutes. Then assert, *"It's my intent to center myself in my core field."* Continue by asserting, *"It's my intent to turn my organs of perception inward on the level of my core field."* Next, assert, *"It's my intent to fill my core field with bliss, prana, and jing."* Take ten minutes to fill your core field with bliss, prana, and jing. Then count from one to five. When you reach the number five, open your eyes and bring yourself out of the exercise. We recommend that you and your family members repeat the exercise regularly for three weeks.

Issue: Body Image Problems

Body image problems can torment a family member and create self-destructive thoughts and feelings that interfere with their relationships and disrupt their self-esteem. Body image problems usually emerge when a child's search for a stable personal identity begins to dominate their lives. For most children, this transition takes place between their sixth and seventh year, the same time they begin school. Although the problem can begin in the home, it's often made worse by the taunting of other children.

Our work with Denise and her parents, Frank and Mara, will illustrate how important it can be for a child—or any family member, regardless of their gender and age—to have a positive body image. Denise was six and exceptionally tall for her age when her parents consulted us. Because of her size, most people thought she was older and therefore more developed. As a result, they had expectations that she was unable to meet. Her father, Frank, compounded the problem by constantly saying that she was too big for her age. The issue simmered on the back burner until Denise started school. Then it came to a boil because of the insensitivity of her teacher and the taunting of her classmates, who began to call her "giraffe."

We explained to Frank and Mara that Denise's body image problem had created blockages in her first and second chakras—and that the two kwas had also been affected.

The condition of the first chakra affects a person's sense of security and body image. The condition of the second chakra affects a person's level of vitality and gender orientation. The two kwas also have a significant influence on body image because they provide a person with the prana they need to experience physical pleasure.

Solution: To help Denise overcome her body image problem, we taught her parents to perform two exercises. We recommend that you perform the same exercises with your child for at least two weeks or until they're comfortable performing them alone.

In the first exercise, you and your child will activate and center yourselves in your first and second chakra fields. Then you will fill both chakra fields and the two kwas with prana.

After you've performed the first exercise for two weeks, you can help your child enjoy their body on both the physical and non-physical levels by teaching them to perform the Self-Love Meditation.

It's their subtle field which supplies your children with joyful and satisfying feelings and sensations. Children and adults who experience their subtle field and the joyful feelings and sensations that emerge from it rarely develop long-term body image problems.

We recommend that you perform the exercise with your child for two weeks. After that, your child can perform the exercise on their own.

An adult who suffers from a body image problem should perform both exercises alone until the issue no long disturbs them.

Denise's parents followed our instructions. Frank stopped making comments about his daughter's size and instead encouraged her to participate in sports where her size would be an advantage. Because of his support, she began to play field hockey and quickly became a valuable member of a local team. He also taught Denise to perform the First and Second Chakras—Two Kwas Meditation and the Self-Love Meditation. Denise and her father practiced both meditations regularly and, by the time they'd completed the process, Denise's body image had improved dramatically. By performing these exercises with your child, you can expect the same results.

Exercise: First and Second Chakras— Two Kwas Meditation

We recommend that you teach this exercise to your child and practice it with them. You can also practice this exercise on your own if you suffer from a body image problem.

To begin the meditation, find a comfortable position with your back straight. Close your eyes and breathe deeply through your nose for two to three minutes. Then count backward from five to one and from ten to one. Continue by asserting, *"It's my intent to go to my personal healing space."* Then bring your awareness to your body, soul, and spirit. Enjoy your healing space for five minutes. Then assert, *"It's my intent to activate my first chakra."* Continue by asserting, *"It's my intent to center myself in my first chakra field."* Enjoy the shift for two to three minutes. Then assert, *"It's my intent to fill my first chakra field with prana and jing."* Take five minutes to complete the process. Then assert, *"It's my intent to activate my second chakra."* Continue by asserting, *"It's my intent to center myself in my second chakra field."* Take a few moments to enjoy the shift. Then assert, *"It's my intent to fill my second chakra field with prana and jing."* Take five minutes to complete the process. Then assert, *"It's my intent to fill my right and left kwas with prana and jing."* Continue to fill the two kwas with prana and jing for another five minutes. Then count from one to five. When you reach the number five, open your eyes and bring yourself out of the meditation.

We recommend that you practice the exercise with your child every day for two weeks. After that you can move on to the Self-Love Meditation.

EXERCISE: The Self-Love Meditation

We recommend that you teach this exercise to your child and practice it with them. You can also practice this exercise on your own if you suffer from a body image problem.

To begin the Self-Love Meditation with your child, find a comfortable position with your back straight. Close your eyes and breathe deeply through your nose for two to three minutes. Then count backward from five to one and from ten to one. Continue by asserting, *"It's my intent to go to my personal healing space."* Then bring your awareness to your body, soul, and spirit. Enjoy your healing space for five minutes. Then assert, *"It's my intent to visualize a screen eight feet (two and a half meters) in front of me."* Continue by asserting, *"It's my intent to visualize myself on the screen."* As soon as your image appears on the screen, assert, *"It's my intent to radiate love from my human heart to the image of myself on the screen."* Continue by asserting, *"It's my intent to radiate prana and jing in the form of unconditional love from my heart chakra to the image of myself on the screen."* Then assert, *"It's my intent to radiate transcendent love from my third heart, Atman, to the image of myself on the screen."* Enjoy the process for five minutes. Then assert, *"It's my intent that my image on the screen radiates love from all three hearts back to me."* Take ten minutes to experience the flow of love. Then release your image and the visual screen. Continue by counting from one to five. When you reach the number five, open your eyes. You'll feel wide awake, perfectly relaxed, and better than you did before.

Continue to perform the exercise with your child until they no longer are disturbed by a body image problem.

Issue: Mobbing and Bullying

In the ethnology of bird behavior, mobbing takes place when large numbers of one species mob one or more members of another species that has been perceived to be a threat. In human interactions, mobbing occurs when a group of people "go after" a person because they are perceived to be different—and their behavior and/or beliefs have been judged by the group to be unacceptable.

People who participate in mobbing spread rumors and use threats as well as satire and sarcasm to isolate and intimidate another peron. Although mobbing is often compared to bullying, mobbing always involves a group. It also has another dimension to it that can make it more threatening. While bullying can be carried out by one person who is jealous, envious, or simply needs an outlet for their aggression, the goal of mobbing is to make a child or adult suffer—and to create an intolerable environment for them.

The psychological and physical violence that results from either mobbing or bullying can have lasting effects on both adults and children. Even the threat of psychological or physical violence can traumatize a child or adult by creating blockages that prevent them from expressing themselves freely and developing and/or maintaining a healthy self-image. People of any age who've been the target of mobbing or bullying frequently suffer from adjustment disorders, headaches, depression, skin diseases, and digestive disorders. Most if not all of these symptoms can have their foundation in subtle, energetic projections and trauma scars, which can disrupt the flow of subtle energy through the targets subtle field.

Solution: Since it's difficult to stop other people from behaving badly, you must do whatever is possible to enhance your family members' inner strength and self-esteem in order to minimize the problem.

To do that, you can teach them to perform the Self-Esteem Mudra and Empowerment Mudra. If your child is a target, perform both mudras with them every day for at least two weeks. If it's an adult family member who has been targeted, we recommend that they perform the mudras for two weeks on their own.

After two weeks, you can begin to locate and release the blockages and trauma scars created by mobbing or bullying. An adult family member should continue to perform the mudras on their own after the blockages and trauma scars have been released. A child should continue to perform the mudra with a parent so that they will be fortified against the violence and psychological attacks that can accompany mobbing or bullying.

EXERCISE: The Self-Esteem Mudra

Perform the Self-Esteem Mudra (see figure 16: The Self-Esteem Mudra, page 141) on your own or with your child regularly, along with the Empowerment Mudra.

EXERCISE: The Empowerment Mudra

The Empowerment Mudra is designed to transform prana into personal power—and to distribute it uniformly throughout your subtle energy field.

You can perform the mudra with your child if they've been the target of mobbing or bullying, or on your own if you've been the target.

To begin, find a comfortable position with your back straight. Then place the tip of your tongue directly behind the point where your teeth meet your upper gum. Put the outside tips of your thumbs together to form a triangle. Then put the tips of your index fingers together to form the second triangle. Once the tips of your index fingers are touching, put the outside of your middle and ring fingers together, from the first to the second joint. Then put the inside tips of your pinkies together to form a third triangle.

When you look down at your hands, you will see three triangles. The first triangle has been created by your thumbs. The second triangle has been created by your index fingers, and the third triangle has been created by your pinkies (see figure 26: The Empowerment Mudra).

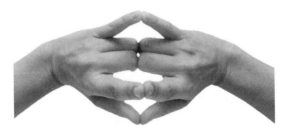

Figure 26: The Empowerment Mudra

Hold the mudra for ten minutes with your eyes closed. After ten minutes, release it. Then count from one to five. When you reach the number five open your eyes and bring yourself out of the exercise.

Releasing Negative Projections

Intimidation, physical violence, and mobbing will always be accompanied by projections of distorted energy. In fact, it's projections on the subtle level that can have the most negative long-term effects. To counteract those effects, it's essential to release the distorted fields. After they've been released, you can release the trauma scars that accompany them. To release negative projections, you will use the prana box. Since most negative projections come in the form of cords, attachment fields, and clinging fields, you can use the techniques you learned in chapter 16 to release them.

Exercise: Releasing Trauma Scars

By using the prana box to release traumas scars, you will remove the legacy of psychological and physical violence that normally accompanies mobbing and bullying. To release one or more trauma scars, go to chapter 12. The process is fundamentally the same, except that—this time—you will visualize an image of your child on your screen if they've been the target of mobbing or bullying.

Issue: Childhood Sexuality

Sexuality is much more than sex. It includes values, attitudes, feelings, and social interactions. Sexual development is one part of sexuality. It begins as soon as the child is born. Sexuality is another part. Both have an influence on how a child relates to other people. Infants and children may not think about sexuality in same way as adults, but they learn and interpret messages related to sexuality that will shape their future attitudes and relationships. One issue that can arise very early in a child's development is the creation of sexual inhibitions.

We recognize that different cultures and subcultures can have different sexual norms. However, for a child or any family member to develop a healthy relationship to their own sexuality and to adult sexual relationships, they must be able—at the appropriate times—to spontaneously experience sexual pleasure.

Solution: To help a family member to experience sexual pleasure spontaneously and to prevent sexual inhibitions from disrupting your child's sexual development, you can perform two exercises. The first will enhance the flow of prana and jing through a person's microcosmic circuit. The second will enhance the flow of prana and jing through their right and left kwas.

For children under six, you can use the Visual Screen to perform the exercises. You can teach children older than six the techniques so that they can perform the exercises along with you—or, if they prefer, on their own.

EXERCISE: Microcosmic Circuit Meditation

To perform the Microcosmic Circuit Meditation for yourself, see page 108. To begin the meditation with your child, find a comfortable position with your back straight. Then close your eyes and breathe deeply through your nose for two to three minutes. Continue by asserting, *"It's my intent to go to my personal healing space."* Then bring your awareness to your body, soul, and spirit. Enjoy your healing space for five minutes. Then place the tip of your tongue at the top of your mouth just behind your teeth. This is known as closing the gate. Continue by asserting, *"It's my intent to create a visual screen eight feet* (two and a half meters) *in front of me."* As soon as the screen appears, assert, *"It's my intent to create an image of* (child's name) *on the screen."* Take a moment to observe your child's condition on both the physical and subtle levels. Then assert, *"It's my intent to bring my mental attention to the back of* (child's name)*'s first chakra gate at the base of their spine"* (see figure 13: The Microcosmic Circuit, page 103). Once your mental attention is centered on the back of their first chakra gate, breathe into the back of the gate. Continue to breathe into it for one to two minutes. Then breathe normally again and move your mental attention slowly upward until it reaches the back of their second chakra gate. When it has reached the back of the chakra gate, assert, *"It's my intent to center my mental attention in the back of* (child's name)*'s second chakra gate."* Breathe into the back of the second chakra gate for one to two minutes. Continue in the same way by activating the back of their third, fourth, fifth, sixth, and seventh chakras.

After you've activated the masculine gate of your child's seven traditional chakras, continue by asserting, *"It's my intent to bring my mental attention to the front of* (child's name)*'s seventh chakra gate at the crown of their head."* Once your mental attention is centered on the front of their seventh chakra gate, breathe into it for one to two minutes. Then move your mental attention slowly down the conceptual meridian until you reach the feminine pole of the sixth chakra gate, which is located by their brow. Breathe into it for one to two minutes. Then continue the process, in the same way, until you've activated the feminine gate of their seven traditional chakras.

Once you've activated the front of the seven traditional chakras, assert, *"It's my intent to fill* (child's name)*'s seven chakra fields with prana and jing."* Give them ten minutes to enjoy the experience. After ten minutes, release the screen and the image of your child. Then count from one to five. When you reach the number five, open your eyes and bring yourself out of the meditation. Repeat as needed.

EXERCISE: Energizing the Two Kwas

To begin the exercise, find a comfortable position with your back straight. Then close your eyes and breathe deeply through your nose for two to three minutes. Continue by asserting, *"It's my intent to go to my personal healing space."* Then bring your awareness to your body, soul, and spirit. Enjoy your healing space for five minutes. Then assert, *"It's my intent to create a visual screen eight feet* (two and a half meters) *in front of me."* As soon as the screen appears, assert, *"It's my intent to create an image of* (child's name) *on the screen."* Take a moment to observe your child's condition on both the physical and subtle levels. Then assert, *"It's my intent to fill* (child's name)*'s right and left kwas with blue chi."* Give your child ten minutes to enjoy the process. After ten minutes, release the screen and the image of your child. Then count from one to five. When you reach the number five, open your eyes and bring yourself out of the meditation. Repeat as needed.

Issue—Lack of Self-Esteem

Self-esteem is so obvious to people who have it that its importance is rarely appreciated. For children and adults who lack self-esteem, however, existence can become a constant struggle. Fortunately, with what you've learned so far, you can free yourself or another family member from this self-limiting pattern so that they can enjoy their life and reach their full potential.

Solution: Self-esteem is directly connected to two things: self-confidence and inner joy. To increase self-confidence and inner joy, you (or they) will activate your first, third, and fifth chakras. Then you (or they) will fill all three chakra fields with prana and jing. For children under six, we recommend that you use the Visual Screen to activate your child's chakras and fill them with prana and jing. If your child is older than six, teach them to perform the First, Third, and Fifth Chakra Meditation so that they can perform it along with you or, if they prefer, they can perform it on their own.

We recommend that you perform the exercise regularly, for at least two weeks. After that, you can teach your child to perform the Self-Esteem Mudra (see page 247). Once you've taught your child the mudra, you can perform it along with them—or they can perform it on their own. In either case, continue to perform the mudra until your child's self-esteem has been fully restored.

Exercise:
First, Third, and Fifth Chakra Meditation

To perform the exercise for a child, find a comfortable position with your back straight. Breathe deeply through your nose for two to three minutes. Then count backward from five to one and from ten to one. Continue by asserting, *"It's my intent to go to my personal healing space."* Then bring your awareness to your body, soul, and spirit. Enjoy your healing space for five minutes. Then assert, *"It's my intent to create a visual screen two and a half meters in front of me."* Continue by asserting, *"It's my intent to visualize* (child's name) *on the screen."* Once your child appears, take a few moments to observe their condition on the physical and subtle levels. Then assert, *"It's my intent to activate* (child's name)*'s first chakra."* Continue by asserting, *"It's my intent to fill* (child's name)*'s first chakra field with prana and jing."* Take two to three minutes to enjoy the process. Then assert, *"It's my intent to activate* (child's name)*'s third chakra."* Continue by asserting, *"It's my intent to fill* (child's name)*'s third chakra field with prana and jing."* After another two to three minutes, assert, *"It's my intent to activate* (child's name)*'s fifth chakra."* Then assert, *"It's my intent to fill* (child's name)*'s fifth chakra with prana and jing."* Continue to fill all three fields with prana and jing for ten more minutes. Then release the image of your child and the screen and count from one to five. When you reach the number five, open your eyes and bring yourself out of the meditation.

To perform the exercise for yourself, visualize yourself on the screen and fill your chakra fields with prana and jing.

EXERCISE:
The Self-Esteem Mudra

To perform the Self-Esteem Mudra, see page 141. Practice the mudra on your own or with your child after you've performed the First, Third, and Fifth Chakra Meditation. Continue until you or your child no longer suffers from a lack of self-esteem.

— EIGHTEEN —

Empty-Nesters

By practicing what you've learned in this book, you've been able to heal family relationships and enhance the joy and satisfaction you can share with your family members. However, once your children are ready to create their own homes and families, you will face new and sometimes unexpected challenges.

Of course, the challenges will be easiest to overcome if you've prepared yourself and your family members for them beforehand. We've found that the most effective way to do that is to help your children develop a respect for energy with universal qualities as well as a strong and authentic identity. It's also helpful to recognize that once your children have left the nest, your responsibilities as a parent and spouse must be redefined. For many of you, this will mean recommitting yourself to your partner and to your unfinished spiritual work. It can also mean letting your children go on the subtle levels of energy and consciousness.

Letting Your Children Go

The best thing you can do for your children, when they come of age, is to give them the space they need to be themselves and to follow their life path. This is not a twenty-first-century concept. As early as the sixth century BCE, the Buddha taught his followers that the root of all human suffering is attachment. It's essential to integrate this concept into your life when your children are ready to leave the nest—otherwise you may open the door to disappointment, resentment, and even estrangement.

Natalie consulted us a few days after she returned from her honeymoon with Henry, whom she'd met in Seattle and married a year later. Natalie told us that her twenty-year-old daughter, Elaine, was leaving for college in the fall and that she was having difficulty letting her go. She explained that, since she had divorced Elaine's father, she worried about her all the time. We checked her subtle field and immediately recognized that the problem was caused by attachment fields that she had projected at Elaine, especially during the contentious divorce proceedings, which took place when Elaine was seven years old. Another problem was Natalie's overbearing attitude which had alienated her daughter and had made it increasingly difficult for Natalie to voice her concerns.

To overcome her problem, we taught Natalie to release the attachment fields that she'd projected. Then we brought Elaine and Henry into the process and taught the family to create the mutual field of empathy and to perform the Radiant Tao Meditation. After they'd performed the exercises for two months, they rented a sailboat and sailed around Puget Sound together for several weeks. We received an email after their excursion and learned that it had been a great success and that Elaine was on her way to Paris to study.

Letting your children go is a two-part process. The first part is facilitating your child's individuation. This is an ongoing process that takes place while they're still dependent on you. The process of individuation will provide your children with a life-affirming identity, good character, and a respect for energy with universal qualities.

The second part is letting your adult children go at the appropriate time— while retaining a loving, intimate relationship with them.

If you and your partner have integrated the practices in this book into your lives, then you've already met the first condition. To help you meet the second condition, we've provided you with two exercises that have proven useful to many families. In the first exercise, you will create the mutual field of empathy. We designed this exercise specifically to enhance the empathy family members have for one another. In the second exercise, called the Radiant Tao Meditation, you will strengthen the bonds of love and intimacy that you share with your partner and children.

By performing both exercises when your grown children are ready to leave the nest, you will be able to sustain a healthy relationship with them that will endure as long as you live.

EXERCISE: Creating the Mutual Field of Empathy

Creating the mutual field of empathy will enhance empathy between family members and ensure that they can share their feelings and emotions with each other effortlessly.

In chapter 6, you learned to enhance your empathy for yourself and your family members. In this exercise, you will take empathy one step further by creating the mutual field of empathy. To do that, you and your family members will sit in a circle facing one another. Then you will center yourselves in your collective fields of empathy, fill them with prana, jing, and consciousness, and radiate it all through the mutual field of empathy to your loved ones. Once you've created the mutual field of empathy, it will remain intact and will continue to nourish you regardless of your distance from one another.

To begin, find a comfortable position facing your partner and children. Close your eyes and breathe deeply through your nose for two to three minutes. Then count backward from five to one and from ten to one. Use the Orgasmic Bliss Mudra to bring bliss into your conscious awareness (see figure 9: The Orgasmic Bliss Mudra, page 70). Then hold the mudra and assert, *"It's my intent to center myself in my collective field of empathy."* Continue by asserting, *"It's my intent to turn my organs of perception inward on the levels of my collective field of empathy."* Take a moment to enjoy the shift. Then assert, *"It's my intent to fill my collective field of empathy with prana, jing, and pure consciousness."* Take two to three minutes to enjoy the process. Then assert, *"It's my intent to create a mutual field of empathy—and to share the prana, jing, and consciousness that supports it with my family members assembled here."* Take fifteen minutes to enjoy the process. Then release the mudra and count from one to five. When you reach the number five, open your eyes and bring yourself out of the meditation.

Once you've created the mutual field of empathy, you can take the next step by performing the Radiant Tao Meditation. The Radiant Tao Meditation will gently release any lingering attachments that interfere with your relationship to your children.

EXERCISE: The Radiant Tao Meditation

Parents can perform the exercise together or separately when one of their children is ready to leave the nest. To begin the exercise, close your eyes and breathe deeply through your nose for two to three minutes. Then count backward from five to one and from ten to one. Continue by asserting, *"It's my intent to go to my personal healing space."* Then bring your awareness to your body, soul, and spirit. Enjoy your healing space for five minutes. Then assert, *"It's my intent to create a visual screen eight feet* (two meters) *in front of me."* As soon as the screen appears, assert, *"It's my intent to visualize* (child's name) *and me on the screen bathing in the vitalizing water of the Tao."* The Tao is often symbolized as a river of pure life-affirming water. Using this symbol will enhance the effect of this exercise. Continue by asserting, *"It's my intent that* (child's name) *and I absorb the Tao's life-affirming energy and that it replaces the self-limiting attachments we have to one another."* Take ten minutes to enjoy the process. Then count from one to five. When you reach the number five, open your eyes and bring yourself out of the meditation. Practice the exercise regularly until all remaining attachments are released. (This exercise can be performed next to a natural body of water).

Keeping Love Alive

After many years of being together, familiarity, the addition of children, and projections with individual qualities can disrupt the relationship parents have with one another. In the following pages, we will provide you with three exercises that will restore human love and unconditional love if they have been blocked over time. Both forms of love are important because a healthy partnership is a synthesis of them both.

Human love is influenced by soul vibration, shared core values, and sexual attraction; which is a function of elemental compatibility. Unconditional love is influenced by energy with universal qualities and bliss.

You and your partner can enhance your personal love by performing the following exercise. After that, you and your partner can enhance the unconditional love you can share with one another by performing the Third Heart Field Meditation and the Unconditional Love Meditation.

EXERCISE: Enhancing Human Love

To enhance the amount of human love you can share with your partner, you will center yourself in your reflection centers. Reflection centers are two centers of awareness in the back of your head, just below and on each side of the Eye of Brahma (see figure 27: The Two Reflection Centers, page 254). Then you will fill your right and left armpit cavities with chi. Once you can feel your armpit cavities glowing with energy, you will center yourself in your heart chakra field. Then you will share the excess energy, radiating into your heart chakra field from your armpit cavities, with your partner.

In this exercise, you and your partner will sit eight feet (two and a half meters) apart, facing each other. To begin the exercise, close your eyes and breathe deeply through your nose for two to three minutes. Then count backward from five to one and from ten to one. Continue by asserting, *"It's my intent to center myself in my reflection centers in the back of my head."* Enjoy the shift for five minutes. Then assert, *"It's my intent to center myself in my two armpit cavities."* After two to three minutes, assert, *"It's my intent to fill my two armpit cavities with chi and jing."* Enjoy the process for five minutes more. Then assert, *"It's my intent to fill my heart chakra field with chi and jing radiating from my armpit cavities."* Once the chakra begins to glow with energy, assert, *"It's my intent to share the chi and jing radiating through my heart chakra field with my partner."* Enjoy the process along with your partner for ten minutes more. Then count from one to five. When you reach the number five, open your eyes and bring yourself out of the meditation. Practice the exercise with your partner every day for at least a month. Then perform the exercise whenever you want to give your love life an extra boost.

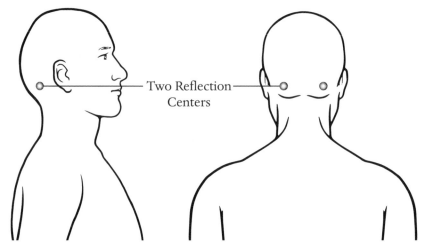

Figure 27: The Two Reflection Centers

Enhancing Unconditional Love

To enhance unconditional love, you will perform two exercises. The first is called the Third Heart Field Meditation. In this exercise, you will enhance your experience of unconditional love. The second exercise is called the Unconditional Love Meditation. In this exercise, you will enhance your ability to share unconditional love in the form of bliss with your partner. Unlike human love, which is a manifestation of energy, unconditional love is a form of consciousness that radiates through your third heart field.

Your third heart field is a resource field that radiates bliss into your conscious awareness from Atman, on the right side of your chest.

EXERCISE: The Third Heart Field Meditation

To begin the exercise, find a comfortable position with your back straight. Close your eyes and breathe deeply through your nose for two to three minutes. Then count backward from five to one and from ten to one. Perform the Orgasmic Bliss Mudra next (see figure 9: The Orgasmic Bliss Mudra, page 70).

Continue to hold the mudra while you assert, *"It's my intent to center myself in my third heart field."* Continue by asserting, *"It's my intent to turn my organs of perception inward on the level of my third heart field."* Take two or three minutes to enjoy the shift. Then assert, *"It's my intent that bliss radiates freely through my third heart field."* Take ten more minutes to enjoy the exercise. Then release the mudra and count from one to five. When you reach the number five, open your eyes and bring yourself out of the meditation.

Perform the exercise for at least seven days or until you feel that bliss radiates freely through your third heart field.

EXERCISE: Unconditional Love Meditation

To begin the exercise, sit facing your partner at a distance of eight feet. Then close your eyes and breathe deeply through your nose for two to three minutes. Count backward from five to one and from ten to one. Then perform the Orgasmic Bliss Mudra (see figure 9: The Orgasmic Bliss Mudra, page 70). Hold the mudra for five minutes. Then continue to hold it while you assert, *"It's my intent to center myself in my third heart field."* Once you're centered, assert, *"It's my intent to turn my organs of perception inward on the level of my third heart field."* Take two to three minutes to enjoy the shift. Then assert, *"It's my intent to fill my third heart field with bliss."* Enjoy the changes you feel for two to three minutes more. Then open your eyes and gaze at your partner.

You and your partner should continue to gaze at one another, while you both assert, *"It's my intent to freely radiate unconditional love from my third heart."* Take ten more minutes to share bliss in the form of unconditional love with your partner. Then release the Orgasmic Bliss Mudra and count from one to five. When you reach the number five, open your eyes and bring yourself out of the exercise. Practice the exercise every day with your partner until unconditional love has transformed the relationship you have with one another.

Creating a New Identity

Even if parents can share human and unconditional love freely with one another, adjusting to life as an empty-nester can be difficult. That's because, over the years, their identities have been influenced by the needs of their children. However, to enjoy life as an empty-nester, creating a new identity based on the needs of an older person with experience and enhanced wisdom is essential.

As you recall, Andrew's mother, Patricia, had projected at him when he was a child in order to enhance his security and make him feel safe.

Unfortunately, Patricia's projections had made it difficult for her to let Andrew go and to establish a healthy identity after he left the nest.

In the process of healing his family dynamic, Andrew had released his attachments to his mother and he'd begun to share life-affirming energy with her. To help Patricia restore her subtle field and to create a life-affirming identity as an empty-nester, we taught her to perform the Identity Fulfillment Meditation.

To perform the exercise she began by centering herself in the Eye of Brahma. Then she filled her three domains with bliss and looked inward on the level of her domains.

If you perform the exercise for at least a month like Patricia did, you will recognize who you are stripped of all your attachments. That will provide you with the flexibility and space you need to create a new identity based on your experience and knowledge.

EXERCISE: Identity Fulfillment Meditation

To begin the meditation, find a comfortable position with your back straight. Then close your eyes and breathe deeply through your nose for two to three minutes. Count backward from five to one and from ten to one. Then use the Orgasmic Bliss Mudra to bring bliss into your conscious awareness (see figure 9: The Orgasmic Bliss Mudra, page 70). Continue to hold the mudra while you assert, *"It's my intent to center myself in my Eye of Brahma."* Enjoy the shift for five minutes. Then assert, *"It's my intent to fill my three domains with bliss."* Continue by asserting, *"It's my intent to turn my appropriate organs of per-*

ception inward on the levels of my light body domain, self-domain, and universal domain." Enjoy the process for ten minutes. Then release the mudra and count from one to five. When you reach the number five, open your eyes and bring yourself out of the meditation.

We recommend that you perform the meditation on a regular basis until you feel entirely comfortable with your new identity.

Patricia performed the exercise for several months. Eventually, we lost touch with her. However, we received a letter from Andrew about six months later. He explained that he and his mother continued to use the techniques they learned from us and that they both continued to benefit from them.

Growing Old Gracefully

In our work, we've found that some empty-nesters blame themselves for the mistakes they made in their youth and as parents, while others blame people who they believe interfered with their life and significant relationships. However, to grow old gracefully, a parent must give up blame in its two forms so that they can find peace and live in the present rather than in the past.

There are two forms of blame. The first form of blame is regret for personal mistakes, which is internalized blame. The second form is resentment for the actions or inaction of people, which is externalized blame. Both disrupt love, intimacy, and the satisfaction that is the product of a life well lived. Fortunately, we've learned through our work that regret and resentment can only oppress a person whose authentic will and desire have become too weak to oppose them.

If regret is interfering with your life as a senior, you can overcome the problem by performing the following two exercises. In the first exercise, you will make a list of regrets that continue to disturb you. Then you will use the bliss box to release the distorted fields that support them. These fields will be located in the sections of your core field associated with will and desire. Each time you release a distorted field from your core field, you will fill the space it occupied with bliss and prana.

In the second exercise, you will overcome any remnant of regret by performing the exercise to overcome blame.

Exercise: Overcoming Regrets

To begin the process, find a comfortable position with your back straight. Then close your eyes and breathe deeply through your nose for two to three minutes. Count backward from five to one and from ten to one. Then assert, *"It's my intent to center myself in my field of will."* Continue by asserting, *"It's my intent to turn my appropriate organs of perception inward in my field of will."* Take two to three minutes to enjoy the shift. Then use the Orgasmic Bliss Mudra to bring bliss into your conscious awareness (see figure 9: The Orgasmic Bliss Mudra, page 70). Continue to hold the mudra while you assert, *"It's my intent to surround the most distorted field in my field of will with a bliss box."* Then assert, *"It's my intent to fill the bliss box with bliss and release the distorted field within it."* Don't do anything after that. The distorted field will be released automatically. Once the distorted field has been released, assert, *"It's my intent to fill my field of will with bliss and prana."* Continue for five minutes more. Then release the bliss mudra and count from one to five. When you reach the number five, open your eyes and bring yourself out of the meditation.

Continue to perform the exercise regularly, always releasing the most distorted field, until there are no longer any distorted fields left in your field of will that support regrets. Then perform the same exercise in your field of desire until there are no longer any distorted fields left that support regrets. Once you've released all the distorted fields that supported regrets, you can enhance your condition even further by performing the technique to overcome self-blame.

Exercise: Technique to Overcome Blame

To begin the exercise, find a comfortable position with your back straight. Breathe deeply through your nose for two to three minutes. Then count backward from five to one and from ten to one. Continue by asserting, *"It's my intent to go to my personal healing space."* Then bring your awareness to your body, soul, and spirit. Enjoy your healing space for five minutes. Then assert, *"It's my intent to activate my first chakra."* Continue by asserting, *"It's my intent to center myself in my first chakra field."* Next, assert, *"It's my intent to activate my third chakra."* Continue by asserting, *"It's my intent to center myself in my third chakra field."* Take a few moments to enjoy the shift; then assert, *"It's my intent to fill my first and third chakra fields with prana."* Take five minutes to enjoy the process. Then assert, *"It's my intent to activate my energy center in my right sole."* Continue by asserting, *"It's my intent to activate the energy center in my left sole."* After the energy centers in your soles have become active, assert, *"It's my intent that the prana radiating through my first and third chakra fields flows into the energy centers in my soles."* Enjoy the effects for fifteen minutes more. Then count from one to five. When you reach the number five, open your eyes and bring yourself out of the exercise.

If you practice the technique regularly, in a short time, you will be able to enjoy your age without regrets getting in your way.

If you've been prevented from growing old gracefully by resentments, we recommend that you perform the following two exercises.

EXERCISE: Releasing Attachments to People You Resent

We taught the exercises to Abraham's grandmother Azul, who had been diagnosed with advanced cancer. For most of her life, she had resented her father (who had forced her into an arranged marriage) and her husband (who had died in 2001). She spoke with some difficulty, but from our two sessions with her we learned that she never felt that her life was her own.

We stayed in contact with Abraham until Azul's death seven months later. In his last email, we learned that the exercises had helped Azul find the peace she sought and that she died peacefully in the company of her children and grandchildren.

To overcome resentment, you will make a list of people whom you resent. Then you will choose one person from the list. After you've made your choice, you will release the most disruptive cord and/or attachment field that continues to bind you to them.

To begin the exercise, find a comfortable position with your back straight. Then close your eyes and breathe deeply through your nose for two to three minutes. Count backward from five to one and from ten to one. Continue by asserting, *"It's my intent to go to my personal healing space."* Then bring your awareness to your body, soul, and spirit. Enjoy your healing space for five minutes. Then assert, *"It's my intent to create a visual screen eight feet* (two and a half meters) *in front of me."* As soon as the screen appears, assert, *"It's my intent that* (name of the person you resent) *appears on the screen in front of me."* Then assert, *"It's my intent to become aware of the most disruptive cord or attachment field that connects me to* (name of person you resent)." Take a moment to observe the cord or attachment field.

If it's a cord, it will be long and thin and will extend from your energy field to the person you resent. If it's an attachment field, it will have a long, rectangular shape and will be extremely dense and sticky.

After you've examined the cord or attachment field, assert, *"It's my intent to surround the cord* (or attachment field) *I have in mind with a prana box."* Then assert, *"It's my intent to fill the prana box with prana and to release the cord* (or attachment field) *and its source and extensions."* As soon as the cord (or attachment field) has been released, you will feel a shift in your energetic condition. Pressure will diminish. And the strength of your resentment will decrease.

Continue by releasing the prana box, the image of the person on the screen, and the visual screen. Then take ten minutes to enjoy the effects. After ten minutes, count from one to five. When you reach the number five, open your eyes and bring yourself out of the exercise.

Continue to perform the exercise until all the cords or attachment fields that bind you to the person you resent have been released. Once you've gone through your list and released all the cords and attachment fields that have contributed to your feelings of resentment, you can remove the last remnants of resentment by performing the Five Elements Water Ritual.

EXERCISE: The Five Elements Water Ritual

To perform this ritual, you will need a small piece of a cardboard box (one inch by three inches), one small piece of paper (two square inches), one paper clip, a pinch of flour, and a small piece of duct tape for each resentment you want to permanently release. Write one resentment on each piece of paper. Coat one side of the cardboard with flour. This side will be the deck of your cardboard boat. Then open one end of the paper clip so that it forms a straight point. Pierce the cardboard with the pointed end and use the duct tape to attach your paper to the other end of the paper clip. Once you've prepared each vehicle, go to a body of water, either a stream or lake. Then place the vehicles with your resentments in the water. Once they're in the water, light them so that the cardboard boats and the papers with the resentments burn completely. The close your eyes and assert, *"It's my intent to leave all the resentments I've released and all the energy and consciousness that support them permanently behind me."* Enjoy the meditation for ten minutes more. Then open your eyes and let the lightness you experience radiate through your subtle field and physical-material body.

Conclusion

In this book, you took an exciting journey through inner space. In the process, you discovered that you have the innate power to heal yourself, your family members, and your family relationships.

For many of you, what you've learned is just the beginning of a lifelong journey in personal development and self-realization. By continuing to use what you've learned and by expanding your knowledge and skills, you will continue to enrich your relationship to Universal Consciousness, yourself, and your family members.

Spiritual growth comes from many things, including life-affirming decisions, lifestyle choices, and healthy family relationships. Perseverance in the work of deep family healing is also essential. Continue to use our book and practice what you've learned. By doing that, and by learning more about yourself and your unique place in the universe, you will grow in wisdom and you will become a channel of healing and unconditional love that will make a deep and abiding impact on all the people you know and love.

Glossary

Acupuncture point: A subtle energy point located within a meridian.

Ancestral chi: Chi that is inherited from parents. Ancestral chi cannot be changed or influenced by working on your subtle energy field or by changing your lifestyle.

Ancestral poisons: See poisons of the ancestors.

Appropriate life partner: A person whose soul vibration, core values, and dominant element are compatible with yours.

Armpit cavities: Compliment the functions of the upper dantian. There are two—one on each side of the upper dantian.

Atman: The thumb-sized point on the right side of the chest where universal love in the form of bliss emerges into a person's conscious awareness. By following the Atman inward, a person will become aware of their a priori union with Universal Consciousness.

Attachments: Created when two or more fields with individual qualities bond together within the subtle field. They can disrupt wellness on both the subtle and physical levels in three ways: they can restrict a person's access to prana, they can create restrictive patterns (personality issues), and they can keep a person attached to people and relationship issues that remain unresolved from childhood and/or past lives.

Attachment fields: Projections of energy with individual qualities. They normally have a long, rectangular shape and are extremely dense and sticky.

It's because of these qualities that an attachment field can easily penetrate a person's energy field. The perpetrator's motive for projecting an attachment field, whether they are fully conscious of the projection or not, will be to compel their target to bond with them in an unhealthy way.

Auric fields, auras: Large fields of prana. From the surface of your body on each dimension, your auric fields extend outward (in all directions) from about two inches (six centimeters) to more than twenty-six feet (six and a half meters). Structurally, each auric field is composed of an inner cavity and a thin surface boundary, which surrounds it and gives it its characteristic egg shape.

Authentic desires: Desires that emerge from the authentic mind. Basing decisions and activities on authentic desires will help a person stay centered in their subtle energy field and will enhance the flow of prana through their subtle energy system.

Authentic mind: Composed of the subtle field, the nervous system, and a person's organs of perception, which can be directed at both the external environment (the physical world) and the internal environment (the subtle worlds of energy and consciousness). The authentic mind is a person's authentic vehicle of awareness and expression.

Back-front polarity: The back is masculine in relationship to the front because the movement of masculine energy is strongest through the main masculine meridian, the governor, in the back of the body. The movement of feminine energy is strongest through the main feminine meridian, the conceptual, in the front of the body. Back-front polarity is the same for men, women, and children. It regulates a person's ability to express anger, fear, pain, and joy—the four authentic emotions. It also affects self-confidence, self-esteem, and a person's ability to create and maintain a strong personal identity.

Balance of elements: See elements.

The Bhagavad Gita: A revered Yogic text that teaches that enlightenment can only be achieved when the field of knowledge (the physical and non-physical universe), the knower (the authentic mind), and knowledge (universal energy and consciousness) become one.

Bliss, orgasmic bliss: The most powerful force in the universe. Every human being is in bliss, although most people are unaware of it. According to the Tantrics, orgasmic bliss is an enduring condition deep inside the subtle field created through the union of consciousness (Shiva) and energy (Shakti).

Blockage: Any field of energy or consciousness with individual qualities that disrupts the flow of prana and/or consciousness through a person's subtle field and prevents a person from remaining centered in their authentic mind.

Boundaries: Separate a person's internal environment from the external environment. They are composed of prana in the form of elastic fibers that crisscross each other in every imaginable direction. In the subtle field there are many boundaries, including the surfaces of the auras, chakra fields, and resource fields, as well as the kandas, dantians, and their complimentary cavities.

Buddha, Gautama: A sage who lived in the fifth century BCE. He taught that it was possible to achieve self-realization by embracing a Middle Way between sensual indulgence and severe asceticism.

Chakra(s): Sanskrit word which means "wheel." There are 146 chakras. Each chakra has two parts: a chakra field, which is an immense field of prana; and a gate, which appears as a brightly colored disk that spins rapidly at the end of what looks like a long axle or stalk. Chakras transmit and transmute prana into different frequencies that can be used by the organs and vehicles in the subtle energy field.

Chakra gate: see chakra(s).

Chakra field: Each chakra is composed of a chakra gate and a chakra field. The chakra field is an immense field of prana composed of subtle energy and a surface boundary. The healthier the chakra field, the larger it will be. In most cases a chakra field will extend a significant distance from the surface of a person's body.

Character, good character: The qualities of good character include non-harming, discipline, courage, patience, perseverance, long-suffering, and loyalty. These qualities can be enhanced by a person who brings their subtle energy field into a state of radiant good health.

Chi: A form of non-physical energy with universal qualities that is at the center of family life. When chi flows freely though a family member's subtle field, they will be able to share pleasure, love, intimacy, and joy without restriction.

Consciousness with individual qualities: Creates ideas, thoughts, notions, beliefs, etc., which are in opposition to life-affirming qualities such as compassion, empathy, freedom, and respect for women and children. If enough fields of consciousness with individual qualities become trapped in a person's subtle field, they can contribute to the creation of the individual mind and ego.

Controlling waves: Waves of energy with individual qualities. In most cases, they're projected by a person who seeks to control and/or change an aspect of another person's behavior and/or personality. Controlling waves are normally wedge-shaped when they emerge from the perpetrator's subtle field. Once the controlling wave has entered their target's energy field, it will quickly expand until it fills a large portion of their field.

Cord: A projection of energy with individual qualities in the form of a long, thin cord that is hollow in the center. It's a manifestation of dependency, need, and/or desire that can border on obsession. Cords manifest the perpetrator's desire or need to hold on to or have contact with their target.

Core field: A resource field that contains the sixteen functions of mind, including will, intent, desire, resistance, surrender, acceptance, knowing, choice, commitment, rejection, faith, enjoyment, destruction, creativity, empathy, and love.

Core values: Influence how a person interacts with their partner/other people and how they view the world. A healthy relationship requires that partners share core values that are life-affirming. People with core values that are life-affirming are always compatible because life-affirming core values will do two things: they will support the free radiation of universal feminine energy, and they will support one's purpose for being incarnated in this life.

Dantians: According to Taoist adepts, there are three dantians that are part of a human being's subtle anatomy. They serve as reservoirs of subtle energy and consciousness. The lower dantian is located in the center of the abdomen. Located above it, in the center of the chest, is the middle dantian, and located in the center of the head is the upper dantian.

Dao: See Tao.

Dharma: Comes from the Sanskrit root *dhri*, meaning to "uphold" or to "sustain." Both Yoga and Tantra teach that all human beings share a collective dharma, which is to achieve self-realization. Every human being also has a personal dharma, which is their unique path of healing and personal liberation. By following dharma, a person will learn who they are and what they are capable of achieving in this life.

Distorted energy: Has individual qualities such as color, weight, density, and level of activity. The heavier, darker, and more active the energy's appearance, the more distorted and disruptive it will be. Distorted energy that becomes trapped in a person's subtle field becomes part of the karmic baggage they carry from one life to another.

Domains: A person can experience the world, through their authentic mind, from different perspectives. To an adept, each perspective will look and feel like a large field on the subtle level of consciousness. We call these fields "domains." It's through the perspective of the self-domain that the authentic mind perceives itself and recognizes its eternal relationship to the universe. It's through the perspective of the light body domain that the authentic mind perceives energy with universal qualities, including fields of subtle energy that support pleasure, love, intimacy, and joy. And it's though the perspective of the universal domain that the authentic mind perceives Universal Consciousness and the timeless state of bliss that exists a priori within you.

Dominant element: Each person has one element that dominates their character. When prospective partners have dominant elements that are in harmony, they will have a deep, natural affinity for one another. In most cases, the affinity will be both sexual and spiritual because the partners will be sharing the same outlook on life, which will make the relationship intoxicating for them both.

Elements: The five elements—earth, wood, metal, water, and fire—provide structure and stability in a person's life and relationships. They influence how a person interacts with other people and their physical-material environment.

They also influence character, particularly how disciplined, loyal, patient, and perseverant a person will be. They also influence whether a person is able to maintain their integrity during difficult times (long-suffering) and whether they will refrain from harming people in word, thought, and deed.

Empathy: Empathy is one of the key ingredients of successful relationships because it helps family members understand the perspectives, needs, and intentions of their loved ones. On the subtle levels, every person has three fields of empathy. They're resource fields through which energy can be exchanged selflessly without the "I" or the ego getting in the way. The three fields of empathy are known as the Public Field of Empathy, the Personal Field of Empathy, and the Transcendent Field of Empathy.

Energetic blockage: See blockage.

Energetic projection: Any projection of energy or consciousness with individual qualities. Projections can take the form of cords, controlling waves, and attachment fields. In some cases, they can be accompanied by non-physical beings. When an energetic projection becomes trapped in a person's energy field, it can cause self-limiting and anti-self patterns.

Energetic vehicle: There are two types of energetic vehicles in the human energy field: energy bodies and sheaths. Both are composed of prana. Energy bodies allow a person to be present and to experience the world through intuition, the organs of perception, and the functions of mind. Sheaths allow a person to express themselves and to interact with the world through the organs of expression. Humans have energy bodies and sheaths on all dimensions of the physical and non-physical universe.

Energy bodies: Part of the human energy field. They are composed entirely of energy with universal qualities. Functionally, they allow a person to be present and to function in both the physical and subtle environment via their intuition, organs of perception, and functions of mind.

Energy system: A system of subtle energetic organs. According to Yoga, the energy system is composed of chakras, auric fields, meridians, minor energy centers, kandas, and additional energetic organs that work to maintain a person's well-being. According to Taoism, the energy system includes dantians, subsidiary cavities, meridians, gates, and acupuncture points. The energy system can be thought of as a power plant and grid of substations and power lines that transmute consciousness into prana and prana from one frequency to another.

Energy with individual qualities: Moves in waves or dense fields that have what you can think of as character—or what we call a "flavor." It can accumulate within a person's subtle energy field. Attachments to energy with individual qualities can disrupt the flow of prana through the subtle energy field and can prevent a person from staying centered in their authentic mind.

Energy with universal qualities: Never fundamentally changes. It goes by many names: shakti, prana, chi, etc. It's the energy that is transmitted through the chakras, meridians, and auric fields. It emerges into a person's conscious awareness as pleasure, love, intimacy, and joy, as well as truth, freedom, and bliss.

Enlightenment: A state of permanent bliss. When a person consciously experiences their a priori state of enlightenment, the existential problem of existence disappears, and they experience inner peace.

Environmental chi: A form of energy with universal qualities that a person absorbs directly from the physical or non-physical environment. Environmental chi can be influenced by a person's decisions and interactions with other people, which means it can be enhanced and strengthened.

Ever-present Now: The eternal present; the eternal space/time a person inhabits when they are present in their authentic mind.

External projections: Waves and fields of energy and consciousness with individual qualities that can be projected from one person to another. If a person has become attached to an external projection, it will be integrated into their individual mind and ego and become a part of the karmic baggage they carry in their subtle field.

Eye of Brahma: The inner eye. It's sometimes called the eye of wisdom. While the physical eyes see things in the material world, the Eye of Brahma sees the subtle world where truth can be recognized without the distortion of time and space.

Feminine energy: After emerging from Universal Consciousness, universal feminine energy began to function as the driving force of evolution. It's feminine energy emerging from every corner of the universe and from every female of every species, providing the power to create and procreate. Feminine energy supports love, intimacy, and joy, motivating humans to share intimacy with one another.

Field of empathy: A resource field through which a person can share energy and consciousness without the "I" or the ego getting in the way. The field of empathy has three parts: the Public Field of Empathy, the Personal field of Empathy, and the Transcendent Field of Empathy.

Field of knowledge: The physical and non-physical universe.

Five elements: See elements.

Five Elements Kitchen: One of the cornerstones of Chinese culture. Once the Chinese identified the five elements, they set about categorizing all foods, beverages, and condiments into the five categories. The Five Elements Kitchen will provide you and your family with a balanced diet rich in healthy foods. It will also provide you and your family with enough chi on a daily basis to perform your activities at an enhanced level.

Functions of mind: Each person has within their core field sixteen important functions of mind through which their power, creativity, and radiance emerge. The sixteen functions of mind include intent, will, desire, resistance, surrender, acceptance, knowing, choice, commitment, rejection, faith, enjoyment, destruction, creativity, empathy, and love.

Good character: The principle qualities of character include non-harming, patience, perseverance, discipline, long-suffering, and courage. Energy with universal qualities is both the foundation and product of good character. This means that people who have good character are disciplined, patient, and courageous. They persevere and don't harm other creatures in thought or deed.

Governor meridian: The most important masculine meridian in the human energy field. It connects the chakras below, above, and within body space to one another, and it serves as a boundary for the nine cavities described by the Taoists. Along with the conceptual meridian, it forms the foundation of the microcosmic circuit.

Hatha Yoga: A branch of Raja Yoga that uses asanas (physical exercises), breath control, and proper diet to purify the body and to achieve higher states of consciousness.

Individual mind and ego: If enough fields of energy and consciousness with individual qualities become trapped in a person's subtle field, they can create an individual mind and ego that function in opposition to the authentic mind. The individual mind and ego has two parts: the "I," which creates a false identity; and the ego, which manifests a false personality. Together, they can disrupt a person's ability to be and express themselves freely and engage in life-affirming family relationships.

Individuation: The process of physical and subtle development a child must complete in order to participate in life-affirming family relationships. For a child to successfully individuate, parents must provide them with an environment that fosters a life-affirming identity, good character, and a respect for universal feminine energy

Inner peace: Inner peace is a state of stillness that emerges from deep within a person. It emerges when movement stops and a person can focus their mind on the joy that spontaneously radiates through their subtle field.

Inner vision: Inner vision enables a person to intuitively recognize a compatible life partner. To enhance inner vision, a person can perform the Inner Vision Mudra and the Eye of Brahma Technique.

Inner wisdom: The wisdom that comes from experience and from trusting your own intuition and discernment.

Intent: In deep healing, a person's intent serves the same function as a computer software program. Just as a software program instructs a computer to perform a particular task, the intent will instruct the authentic mind, which is composed of the brain, central nervous system, and a person's non-physical field of energy and consciousness, to locate a concentration of karmic baggage or an attachment that is responsible for a physical ailment or self-limiting pattern.

Inter-dimensional being: Any sentient being that has both physical and non-physical vehicles. Because humans have physical and non-physical vehicles, they are inter-dimensional beings.

Intrusions: Created by the violent projection of energy or consciousness with individual qualities into a person's subtle field, intrusions produce blockages and self-limiting patterns.

Kali Yuga: A time in human history when consciousness remains mired at such a mundane level that there is very little room for family relationships to blossom. During Kali Yuga, honesty and trust are in short supply and relationships are dominated by ego and self-limiting patterns that disrupt love and intimacy.

Kanda: There are three kandas that influence the subtle organs in body space. The first kanda is located behind the first chakra at the base of the spine. The second kanda is located behind the heart chakra, and the third kanda is located behind the back of the crown chakra. The kandas are energetic hubs that transmit prana from resource fields to the organs of the subtle field, particularly the seven traditional chakras and the major meridians that connect them.

Karma: A Sanskrit word that can be translated as activity or action. In the west, karma has been defined as the "cumulative effect of action," which is commonly expressed as "you reap what you sow."

Karmic baggage: Karmic baggage is the accumulated amount of energy and consciousness with individual qualities that a person carries in their subtle field from one lifetime to another. In your subtle field, karmic baggage creates pressure and muscle ache when you're stressed, and it creates self-limiting and anti-self patterns that produce anxiety, self-doubt, and confusion.

Karmic wound: An energetic wound caused by energetic trauma. See karmic baggage.

Karmic pattern: A pattern created by attachments to karmic baggage. A karmic pattern is always self-limiting; given enough time, it will disrupt personal power, creativity, and family relationships.

Knower: A person's authentic mind.

Knowledge: Universal energy and consciousness.

Kundalini-Shakti, Kundalini: The greatest repository of prana in a person's energy field. It comes in two forms: structural Kundalini, which maintains stability and individual identity; and the serpent energy, which is located at the base of the spine and provides power and vitality.

Kwas: Reservoirs of chi located on each side of the lower dantian. The right and left kwas compliment the functions of the lower dantian. It's the support of the kwas that enables a person to fully express pleasure, particularly sexual pleasure.

Lao Tsu: Lived in China in the sixth century BCE. He taught that the physical world was the outer manifestation of a non-physical world of energy and consciousness. According to Lao Tsu and the Taoist adepts who followed him, subtle energy and consciousness serve as the foundation of human awareness and vitality.

Life-affirming identity: Self-confidence, self-esteem, and empathy for others.

Life-affirming qualities: The foundation of a person's power, creativity, and radiance. These qualities include pleasure, love, intimacy, and joy, as well as the qualities of good character. See character.

Life force: Life force is not something you can feel since it emerges from Universal Consciousness, but you can recognize it because it creates a buzz that enlivens your body. You can have a direct experience of life force by centering yourself in Atman on the right side of your heart chakra.

Light body domain: See domains.

Lower dantian: See dantians.

Mantra: A word, sound, or short sentence that a person repeats in order to focus their mind and enter a state of meditation.

Mental attention: A person's mental attention functions simultaneously in all worlds and dimensions in both the physical and non-physical universe. Mental attention can be used to visualize the condition of the subtle field and to release distorted fields of energy and consciousness.

Meridians: Streams of energy that transmit prana from one part of the subtle field to another. The flow of energy with universal qualities through the meridians enables a person to remain centered in their authentic mind, to form an authentic identity, and to participate in transcendent relationships.

Microcosmic circuit: A system of subtle organs that regulates the flow of prana through the subtle energy field. It includes the three dantians and their neighboring cavities as well as the governor and conceptual meridians. It also includes the thirteen chakras in body space because each chakra has important functions related to family relationships and personal well-being.

Middle dantian: See dantians.

Midrashic literature: A genre of rabbinic literature, dating back primarily to the first through tenth centuries, which contains early interpretations and commentaries on the Written and Oral Torah (spoken law and sermons).

Midriff cavities: Compliment the functions of the middle dantian. There are two midriff cavities: the right and left midriff cavities.

Mind: The mind is composed of three essential elements. On the physical level, it includes the brain and nervous system as well as the chemicals in the body, such as hormones that influence its structure and activities. On the non-physical level, the mind includes the subtle field, its organs and vehicles, and the consciousness and prana that nourish them. The combination of physical and non-physical elements creates the third part of the human mind: the network. The network includes the connections the mind has to its individual parts and to things beyond itself. This includes consciousness and energy as well as attachments to other people, non-physical beings, and their projections.

Minor energy centers: These centers are scattered throughout the subtle field. Four principle centers are located in the extremities: one in each hand and one in each foot. Their principle function is to facilitate the movement of prana through the subtle energy field and physical-material body.

Mobbing: In human interactions, mobbing occurs when a group of people go after a person because that person is perceived to be different and their behavior and/or beliefs have been judged to be unacceptable. People who participate in mobbing spread rumors and use threats as well as satire and sarcasm to isolate and intimidate another person. The goal of mobbing is to isolate the person, to make them suffer, and to create an intolerant environment.

Mudra: A symbolic gesture that can be made with the hands and fingers or in combination with the tongue and feet. Each mudra has a specific effect on a person's level of consciousness and the energy flowing through their subtle field.

Muscle testing: Used to test the body's responses when applying pressure to a large muscle. Muscle testing can be used to validate what a person has learned through intuition and discernment. It can provide a person with information about energy blockages, the condition of their organs, nutritional deficiencies, and food allergies.

Mutual field of empathy: A field created by family members that will enhance the empathy they have for one another and ensure that they can share their feelings and emotions effortlessly.

Mutual field of prana: A field created by partners that will be strong enough to prevent karmic baggage and restrictive beliefs from interfering with their experience of intimacy.

Negative ions: Negative ions are created in nature as air molecules break apart due to sunlight, moving air, and water. They're odorless, tasteless, and invisible molecules that we inhale in abundance in certain environments. Think mountains, waterfalls, and beaches. Once they reach our bloodstream, negative ions are believed to produce biochemical reactions that increase the levels of the mood-enhancing chemical serotonin. It's believed that enhanced serotonin levels alleviate depression, relieve stress, and boost energy, all of which can enhance a person's health and relationships.

Non-physical energy: Any form of energy that is located in the non-physical universe.

Non-physical field: See subtle field of energy and consciousness.

Orgasmic bliss: An enduring condition deep within the subtle field created through the union of pure consciousness (Shiva) and energy with universal qualities (Shakti). The merging of consciousness and energy provides a person with a safe haven deep within them where nothing can interfere with their experience of transcendent relationships.

Poisons of the ancestors: These poisons can disrupt a person's well-being as well as their family relationships. To a person with discernment, the poisons look like bundles of long tubes that intrude into the subtle field. Patterns supported by ancestral poisons include depression, self-sabotage, dependency, greed, abusiveness, envy, jealousy, arrogance, and timidity, as well as any other self-limiting pattern that a person inherited from their parents.

Polarity: The degree to which a person's energy field is polarized masculine or feminine. The principle of polarity states that "everything is dual; everything has poles; everything has its pair of opposites; like and unlike are the same; opposites are identical in nature, but different in degree; extremes meet; all truths are but half truths; all paradoxes may be reconciled." There are two polar fields in the physical-material universe. However, in the subtle universe, there are seven.

Prakriti: See Prakriti field.

Prakriti field: The prakriti field is the primordial field of universal feminine energy. It contains some of the highest frequencies of feminine energy. Like all resource fields, the prakriti field fills your energy field and extends beyond it in all directions.

Prana bandage: A prana bandage has a profound impact on a person's psychological health and the health of their energy field. If used correctly, it will seal the energetic wound created by a miscarriage, stillbirth, or abortion.

Purusha: See purusha field.

Purusha field: The primordial field of individual consciousness. It's a resource field that emerged along with the field of prakriti, or the primordial field of feminine energy, during the fourth tattva, or the fourth step in the evolution of the universe.

Reflection centers: Two centers of awareness in the back of the head, just below and on each side of the Eye of Brahma. It's through the reflection centers that a person manifests their authentic identity in the physical and non-physical universe.

Resonance: The mean frequency (vibration) of a field of energy or living being. Every living being and/or field of energy with individual and/or universal qualities has its own unique resonance.

Resource field: A field of consciousness and/or energy with universal qualities that nourishes the subtle field of energy and consciousness and the vehicles within it. Resource fields are almost infinite in size and both fill and surround a person's subtle field on all dimensions.

Restrictive belief: Any belief accepted as true by an institution of society that prevents people from expressing themselves freely. Restrictive beliefs restrict the flow of prana and make it difficult for people to stay centered in their authentic mind.

Restrictive belief system: A manifestion of the individual mind and ego that can restrict consciousness and the flow of prana through a person's subtle field. Restrictive beliefs support self-limiting patterns and behavior. In extreme cases, they will support obsessions, which can lead to anti-self and anti-social behavior.

Reversed polarity: A condition that is caused by an extreme disruption of up-down polarity. Reversed polarity in men will cause the afflicted man to become feminine by his second chakra and masculine by his heart chakra. Reversed polarity in women will cause the afflicted women to become feminine by the heart chakra and masculine by the second chakra.

Self-domain: See domains.

Shakti: See Shiva/Shakti.

Sheaths: Subtle energetic vehicles that interpenetrate the physical-material body and extend a short distance beyond it. They allow a person to interact directly with their external environment and other sentient beings.

Shiva: See Shiva/Shakti.

Shiva/Shakti: Shiva and Shakti are revered as both the divine couple and as the archetypes for consciousness (Shiva) and energy (Shakti). All people have unlimited sources of Shakti's feminine energy (prana-chi) and Shiva's consciousness (Dao) within.

Silver cord: Each energetic vehicle is connected to the subtle field by a silver cord that extends from the back of the neck. The cord can stretch in order to keep the vehicle connected to the subtle field.

Soul vibration: An essential element of compatibility. When partners have compatible soul vibrations, they will feel comfortable with one another, understand one another, and have a strong foundation for intimacy. Soul vibration is determined by many factors, including where a person's soul originated (not all souls originated on earth), how many lives the soul has experienced, where the soul has lived during this life and previous incarnations, and a person's activities and experiences in past incarnations, especially those that were violent and left energetic wounds and trauma scars in their subtle field.

Subtle energy field: Contains energetic vehicles that allow people to express themselves and interact with their environment on both the physical and non-physical levels. It also contains resource fields and a subtle energy system that supplies the subtle field with life-affirming energy.

Subtle energy system: Includes the chakra gates and chakra fields, meridians, auras, and minor energy centers scattered through the subtle energy field as well as the dantians and the smaller cavities, gates, and acupuncture points that compliment them. In the same way that an electrical grid provides energy to homes and businesses, the organs of the subtle energy system transmit and transmute all the prana the physical body and the energetic vehicles need to function healthfully.

Surface boundaries: The surfaces of the energy fields. They surround all of the energy fields (auras and resource fields) and energetic vehicles. A person with weak surface boundaries will feel insecure and won't be able to manifest the qualities of the universal feminine fully.

Tai Chi: An internal Chinese martial art practiced for both its defense training and its health benefits.

Tantra/Tantrics: An ancient school of Indian thought that views energy with universal qualities and consciousness as essentially the same. Shiva, who represents consciousness, and Shakti, who represents energy, were depicted in Tantric iconography in eternal embrace, which means that they are considered ultimately indivisible.

Tao (Dao): The principle that serves as the foundation of the universe. Combined within the Tao are the principles of yin and yang and their manifestations in both the physical-material and subtle universes.

Taoism: A spiritual tradition based on the teachings of Lao Tsu and the Taoist adepts who followed him. Taoism teaches that a person's non-physical field manifests as both a field of energy with universal qualities and a field of pure, life-affirming consciousness.

Tattvas: Steps in the evolutionary process. The word combines the Sanskrit root *tat*, which means "that," and *tvam*, which means "thou" or "you." Thus *tattva* signifies the ancient truth that you are always in union with Universal Consciousness and that you can experience the benefits of union (which include pleasure, love, intimacy, and joy) by remaining centered in your authentic mind. According to Yoga and Tantra, evolution in the physical and non-physical universe has gone through thirty-six tattvas already.

Third heart: See three hearts.

Third heart field: A resource field that radiates bliss into a person's conscious awareness. It's directly connected to Atman, the third heart, on the right side of the chest. It's through the third heart field that a person experiences transcendent relationships with themselves and with the people they love.

Three hearts: Each person has three hearts: the physical heart on the left side of the chest; the heart chakra in the center of the chest; and Atman, the third heart on the right side of the chest. It's from Atman that bliss emerges into a person's conscious awareness.

Transcendence: The state of union or intimacy with Universal Consciousness and one's partner. In the transcendent state, a person can share bliss (on the level of consciousness as well as pleasure) love, intimacy, and joy (on the level of energy) without disruption.

Transcendent relationship: A relationship in which partners can share pleasure, love, intimacy, and joy without blockages, karmic baggage, or anything else getting in the way. Traditional relationship is about living within limitations. In contrast, a transcendent relationship is about transcending limitations.

Trauma: Every traumatic event includes two traumas: a physical trauma, and a subtle energetic trauma that is no less real. The traumas on the subtle levels are responsible for the most acute and enduring symptoms the survivor must endure.

Trauma scar: An energetic trauma that is imprinted in a person's subtle field. A trauma scar looks like a narrow piece of elastic that has been stretched and frozen in place. It will be clear when it's first viewed because it has been suffused with prana. It's only by looking more deeply that a person will notice denser, darker energy in parallel bands running through it. If a trauma scar is left untreated, it can interfere with a person's well-being and family relationships.

Universal Consciousness: The wellspring of bliss. Universal Consciousness combines all aspects of yin-yang. It's the foundation of the authentic mind as well as everything else in the physical and non-physical universe, including time, space, energy, and consciousness.

Universal domain: See domains.

Universal feminine: Motivates humans to unite and to experience intimacy with one another. It makes everybody a healer, a lover, and—on the deepest level—a radiant, transcendent being who has the capacity to transform the world through work and relationships.

Universal feminine energy: See feminine energy.

Universal qualities: Universal qualities include pleasure, love, intimacy, and joy as well as truth and freedom. Universal qualities do not create attachments; they are life-affirming, and they support family relationships.

Up-down polarity: A form of polarity found in the subtle field. In male-female relationships, men are masculine by the second chakra and feminine by the heart chakra. Women are feminine by the second chakra and masculine by the heart chakra. When up-down polarity is in balance, a woman in relationship will be empowered and more self-confident; a man in relationship will become more empathetic, gentle, and receptive to feminine energy.

Upper dantian: See dantians.

Visual screen: With practice, a visual screen will become a reliable tool that can be used to examine the condition of the subtle field during a session of deep healing.

Water cycle: Circulates chi up the back of the body, through the governor meridian, and down the front through the conceptual meridian. The movement of chi in this way enhances intuition and relaxes the nerves along the spine. It integrates the functions of the three dantians, the kwas, the midriff cavities, and the armpit cavities. It distributes chi to the chakras in body space as well as those above and below it.

Wei-Lu gate: Located between the sacrum and the coccyx. It has a direct influence on the kidneys and their ability to function healthfully. According to Chinese medicine, it's where the life force is pumped directly into the subtle energy field.

Yoga: Means "union." It also refers to an ancient scientific method developed in India to achieve enlightenment. Yoga adepts teach that a person's non-physical field manifests as both a field of energy with universal qualities and a field of pure, life-affirming consciousness.

Endnotes

1. Keith Sherwood, *The Art of Spiritual Healing* (revised edition) (Woodbury, MN: Llewellyn Publications, 2016), 27–29.
2. Sherwood, *The Art of Spiritual Healing*, 28-29.
3. Keith Sherwood, *Die Kunst Spiritueller Liebe* (Stuttgart: Luchow Verlag, 2006), 51.
4. Keith Sherwood and Sabine Wittmann, *Energy Healing for Women* (Woodbury, MN: Llewellyn Publicatioons, 2015), 26–27.
5. "Divine madness," Wikipedia, https://en.wikipedia.org/wiki /Divine_madness.
6. "The Whole Body Is the Eye," Chan art and stories, http://www.fgsbmc .org.tw/en/TalesFables.aspx?TFNO=201706020.
7. Sherwood and Wittmann, *Energy Healing for Women*, 71.
8. Sherwood, *The Art of Spiritual Healing*, 105.
9. Keith Sherwood, *Sex and Transcendence* (Woodbury, MN: Llewellyn Publications, 2011), 119.
10. Sherwood, *Sex and Transcendence*, 119–120.
11. Sherwood, *The Art of Spiritual Healing*, 204–206.
12. Sherwood, *The Art of Spiritual Healing*, 220.
13. Keith Sherwood, *Chakra Therapy* (Woodbury, MN: Llewellyn Publications, 1986), 108–109.
14. Sherwood and Wittmann, *Energy Healing for Women*, 196–197.

15. Alexander Kapp, "Protopic: Die Innovation in der Therapie der Atopischen Dermatitis" (Munich 2002), 338.

16. *The Laws of Manu*, 4.173.

17. *The Bible*, Numbers 14:18.

18. Sherwood, *Sex and Transcendence*, 33.

19. Judith S. Wallerstein, PhD, and Julia M. Lewis, PhD, "The Unexpected Legacy of Divorce—Report of a 25-Year Study," *Psychoanalytic Psychology* 21, no. 3 (2004): 353–370. http://citeseerx.ist.psu.edu/viewdoc/download?doi=10.1.1.543.5504andrep=rep1andtype=pdf.

20. Sherwood and Wittmann, *Energy Healing for Women*, 126-127.

21. Rudolf Hänsel, "Die zu häufige Nutzung digitaler Medien vermindert die geistige Leistungsfähigkeit unserer Kinder" (October 2012). http://www.zeit-fragen.ch/index.php?id=1170.

To Write to the Authors

If you wish to contact the author or would like more information about this book, please write to the author in care of Llewellyn Worldwide Ltd. and we will forward your request. Both the author and publisher appreciate hearing from you and learning of your enjoyment of this book and how it has helped you. Llewellyn Worldwide Ltd. cannot guarantee that every letter written to the author can be answered, but all will be forwarded. Please write to:

Keith Sherwood and Sabine Wittmann
℅ Llewellyn Worldwide
2143 Wooddale Drive
Woodbury, MN 55125-2989

Please enclose a self-addressed stamped envelope for reply,
or $1.00 to cover costs. If outside the U.S.A., enclose
an international postal reply coupon.

Many of Llewellyn's authors have websites with additional
information and resources. For more information,
please visit our website at http://www.llewellyn.com

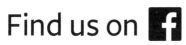
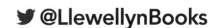

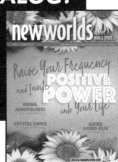

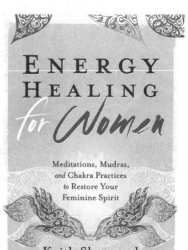

ENERGY
HEALING
for Women

Meditations, Mudras,
and Chakra Practices
to Restore Your
Feminine Spirit

Keith Sherwood
AND Sabine Wittmann
Author of the Bestselling *Chakra Therapy*

Energy Healing for Women
Meditations, Mudras, and Chakra Practices
to Restore Your Feminine Spirit
KEITH SHERWOOD AND SABINE WITTMANN

Reclaim your personal strength, joy, and sense of pleasure through a new understanding of your energy field. *Energy Healing for Women* provides effective exercises to heal injury and restore wholeness on all levels with chakra healing, karmic release, breathwork, massage, mudra, meditation, and affirmation practices.

With each chapter devoted to an energetic issue that may be limiting your power—including difficult issues such as abuse and reproductive wounds—the techniques in this guide will help you feel empowered and improve your courage and vitality. Through story examples, history, theory, and exercises, discover how to:

- Express your feminine energy freely
- Increase your self confidence by fully appreciating and loving your body as it is
- Rise above restrictive beliefs
- Overcome negative archetypes of women and replace them with life-affirming models
- Enhance your intuition, creativity, and sensuality
- Make the transition from a traditional relationship to a transcendent relationship

978-0-7387-4112-3, 264 pp., 6 x 9 $18.99

To order, call 1-877-NEW-WRLD or visit llewellyn.com
Prices subject to change without notice